AGING Culprits!

AGING *Culprits!*

12 MYTHS THAT SABOTAGE YOUR FUTURE AND STEAL YOUR JOY

Eileen Kopsaftis, BS, PT, FAFS, CMI, NE.

Published by Best Seller Publishing®, Pasadena, CA
Best Seller Publishing® is a registered trademark
Printed in the United States of America.
ISBN: 978-1-966395-05-8

For more information, please write:
Best Seller Publishing®
253 N. San Gabriel Blvd, Unit B
Pasadena, CA 91107
or call 1(626) 765 9750
Visit us online at: www.BestSellerPublishing.org

Disclaimer

This information is for educational purposes only. It is not intended to diagnose or treat any medical or health-related conditions. It is not a substitute for medical advice or treatment. Do not disregard professional medical advice or delay treatment because of the information in this book. Discuss your diet with your health care provider prior to making any changes. Please consult with your physician prior to beginning any exercise or self-care program. Have Lifelong Wellbeing, LLC and Eileen Kopsaftis expressly disclaim responsibility, and shall have no liability for any damages, loss, injury, effects, or consequences of any actions taken on the basis of the information provided.

Dedication

To my beloved family, Pete, Robert, Aletia, Sarah, Rebekah, Daniel, Logan, and Luke, who give my life great meaning and motivate me to live well long past 112.

To my wonderful students in the Have Lifelong Wellbeing Academy. This book would not exist if it weren't for them. Every week they inspire me, challenge me, teach me, and give me great joy in training them to age without decline. What other class, with an average age of 70, could do 90 squats in under eight minutes?! They rock!

Contents

INTRODUCTION
Can You Age with Joy?

Jokes abound describing the "golden years," yet if you're spending time in a medical office waiting area several times per month (sometimes per week), it's no laughing matter. Jokes like *I used to do cartwheels but now I tip over while putting on a pair of pants* are very sad comedy. What's so funny about a declining ability to balance on one foot resulting in an increased risk of falls and injury?

Have you heard this one? *The favorite underwear brand of seniors is it depends.* What's funny about unwanted urine leakage?

Or what about the one that advises being kind to your kids because they choose your nursing home? No one ever set a goal to go to a nursing home. Just sayin'.

I have nothing against having a sense of humor, but these jokes are meant to elicit laughter at things that literally suck the joy out of life as you age.

So … if aging has so many things that counter joy, why begin with the question "can you age with joy?" The truth is that the general answer is highly likely to be a resounding NO!

I begin with that question because I believe it IS extremely possible to age with joy.

Let me tell you what you haven't been told.

I've met, and personally worked with, many people over the age of 100. Yes, over 100 years of age! Most of them were still cooking, shopping, driving, cleaning, handling their own finances, and living life large. I know this may not be what is commonly seen, yet it's not as rare as you might think.

The truth is many of the things we see and believe are "caused" by aging are really just myths and misconceptions.

Yes, countless people wear disposable underwear due to unwanted leakage. It's a fact that stores have entire aisles with dozens of brands to choose from. So, how is this a myth? Because it's NOT a rite of passage that you'll need disposable underwear before you can go below ground.

It's a myth because it doesn't have to happen AND it has nothing to do with age.

Surprise!

Common versus Normal

Just because something is common, doesn't mean it's normal. Cardiovascular disease is common, yet it's abnormal functioning of the circulatory system. It's not NORMAL, and it doesn't have to happen, yet it's COMMON.

Whenever you hear "joint pain is normal at your age," aging is then perceived as a loss, a negative, a downward spiral in life. Lifestyle choices are then made based on this perception. Activity is altered, and changes are made in daily life decisions.

But what if it's the perception based on the myth that caused the loss, the negative, the downward spiral?! After all, joint pain is NOT normal despite being commonly experienced by so many people. I've met many people way up there in years who don't experience daily joint pain.

What if busting 12 myths of what's believed about aging and changing the perceptions you hold leads to different lifestyle choices, activities, and daily life decisions?

What if it's all about the actions you take that are a result of a *belief* or *disbelief* in the myths?

Who This Book Is For

This is the right book for you if you want to move away from pain and limited function in daily life, or you simply want to avoid decline, and you're open to making changes that make sense to you so you can age well and enjoy life. Of course, you may be looking for both of those things. That's okay too. You're not just looking for information. You're looking to change your future.

This isn't really the right book for you if you're looking for a magic pill that requires no effort or if you're looking for someone else to "fix" you. There are no shortcuts or magic pills.

How to Get the Most Out of This Book

If you prefer to skip to specific parts of this book to quickly learn what to do without gaining an understanding of why or how to succeed, you're doing a disservice to yourself. You'll gain a depth of understanding of just how much myths and misconceptions have altered life's reality only by reading through each chapter of the book. You'll also learn why solutions you've tried haven't worked as well as what's been shown to work quite well.

If you have specific concerns, you can certainly read those sections first. Because several aspects of common concerns are covered in more than one chapter, this list may be helpful to you:

- Osteoarthritis: chapters 2, 3, 7, 9, and 10
- Osteoporosis: chapters 2, 3, 8, 9, and 10
- Urinary Incontinence: chapters 2 and 5
- Cardiovascular Disease: chapters 2, 3, and 9

Resources on the online *Aging Culprits!* website provide clickable links to movement and exercise videos, articles, and more.

Since you're the only one who can change your life (because no one can do it for you), let's bust some myths and misconceptions and take action!

I'm guilty of substition in our world and I want you to join me. Don't know what substition means? Read on …

PART 1

Misconceptions About Aging

Substition

Ever hear of substition? It's the opposite of superstition. Superstition is something most people believe but isn't true.

Substition is believing something that's utterly true, but yet is disbelieved by most people. You'll find it in an urban dictionary as it was coined by Terry Pratchett in his book, *Making Money*. I haven't read the book, but I first learned the definition of this word from an email I received many years ago. It really resonated with me because I've led a life very often believing in things that are utterly true yet not believed by the general population.

I share this because you'll read many things the general public doesn't believe in the following chapters. Please remember, not believing something doesn't make it not true. A child who wants to play Superman may not believe gravity matters until they jump off the roof of the shed and land splat on the ground. My brother did this when he was four. Not believing or knowing about gravity didn't make gravity not true.

Not believing or knowing about what you'll read in this book doesn't make any of it less true.

I pray that someday soon, everyone will know the truth about aging well. Yes, the myths, misconceptions, and outright superstitions continue to abound about aging, and I'm working to bust them all!

CHAPTER 1

"What Do You Expect at Your Age?" & Other Mindset Mishaps

MYTH: Decline is imminent.

Dr. Jones looked *at me with raised eyebrows when my father answered his question about what medications he was taking. His look said, without saying it, does he have dementia? You see, my dad told the doctor he wasn't on any medications—and my dad was 91 at the time.*

I was used to the doctor's response as health care workers don't tend to see someone my father's age who isn't on any prescription meds. Add to this fact that my dad also had an extensive medical history, including a coronary bypass surgery in his 60s, a coronary stent procedure in his 80s after two heart attacks in a 24-hour period, oral surgery in his 70s due to cancer in the roof of his mouth, and a current diagnosis of chronic lymphocytic leukemia, and it seemed next to impossible that he wasn't on any meds.

I smiled as I informed the man that my father was correct. He was, in fact, not on any medications.

I expect you are wondering how this came about. I'll share that in a bit, but first I want to provide some insights into why the title for this chapter is Mindset Mishaps.

Sources of Mindset Mishaps

We see "age-related this" and "age-related that" diagnosed, written, and reported everywhere in both the health care world and mainstream media. Has that barrage of blaming age for everything from joint damage to losing height ACCELERATED the decline that's seen as so prevalent in our world by creating a destructive mindset?

No, I'm not saying getting older is all in your mind. We all age no matter our efforts to the contrary, but the decline we *expect* is another story. Is mindset the real culprit behind decisions > that determine actions > that lead to decline? Hmmm …

Mindset is defined by *Oxford Learner's Dictionaries* as "a set of attitudes or fixed ideas that somebody has and that are often difficult to change." The doctor mentioned in my father's story had an established set of attitudes about aging and the need for prescription medications. Yes, it's true that medications are a common happenstance in the older population, yet there are many who are not in that category.

I've seen, up close and personal, many people over 100 years old taking no meds for chronic conditions and living lives of quality. They're still driving (safely), cooking, cleaning, shopping, doing their own laundry, handling their own finances, and socializing regularly. However, it appears that the possibility of aging with full function and quality in life SANS medications is unknown to the public.

Why? Is it because mainstream media needs more clicks? After all, more clicks equal more revenue, and they're a profit-driven business. It's reported that the more negative the headlines, the higher the number of clicks that occur.

An analysis of online news headlines found those that include negative words are more likely to draw readers than headlines that do not.[1] Researchers reported a reader was 2.3 percent **more** likely to click on a headline of average length when it contained a *negative* word such as "wrong," "bad," or "awful" than when it contained no emotional words. A reader was also 1 percent **less** likely to click on a headline of average length for each *positive* word it contained.

So … writing about healthy, independent people over the age of 100 doesn't pay the bills?! This disturbing statistic teaches us to be cautious about developing mindsets based on what we read in newspapers and magazine articles because "good, **factual** news" doesn't sell. This includes online media. The fact is there are many, many people aging really well with a high quality of life. You just rarely, if ever, get to read about it.

What is your established set of attitudes about aging? The reason I ask is because they directly impact how you age. Yes, HOW you age. Have you ever met someone who had a really bad attitude? No matter what you told them, it made no difference in what they believed or how they behaved. That's the power of a fixed mindset. The other side of the coin is a growth mindset that seeks truth and alters behaviors based on newfound knowledge.

This doesn't mean it's wise to sway with the wind of every new gimmick, magic herb, or miracle diet. Why?

THERE IS NO MAGIC PILL.

Nonetheless, seeking accurate information and being open to change can make all the difference in the world!

Which mindset do you think would better serve your future self?

A *growth mindset* alters attitudes based on new information. Of course, the new information must come from a reliable source. I'll get to the most important question to ask to help you determine whether a source is trustworthy shortly.

A *fixed mindset* maintains an established set of attitudes and resists change. Often this resistance is so stubborn that no matter how many proven facts are presented, a person may blurt out, "I don't care what the facts are! I refuse to change my mind!"

Studies have shown self-perceptions (mindsets) of aging influence cognitive and physical functioning.[2–4] Those who had more positive self-perceptions at baseline lived seven and a half years longer than those who had a negative self-perception of aging.

Do you have a growth mindset open to learning osteoporosis is technically more of a risk factor than a disease? This diagnosis means there's a risk for fracture. It doesn't mean it will happen. Osteopenia is a risk factor for developing osteoporosis. This means osteopenia is a risk factor for a risk factor. It doesn't mean osteoporosis or fracture will happen.

Do you have a growth mindset open to learning osteoarthritis is not due to wear and tear, compression, or old age? The actual cause of joint damage was determined by the Stanford University School of Medicine and it's NOT old age. Surprised?

Fixed mindsets that believe we age with decline will lead to less activity over time. This then becomes a self-fulfilling prophecy. Job, a familiar biblical character, was known to say, "What I feared most has come upon me."

I'm NOT saying these issues are all in the mind. I AM saying your perception and beliefs around aging will impact the decisions you make about exercise, daily activities, recreation choices, and even the home you buy. Do you know how many people buy a home without stairs, literally **preparing to decline**?!

It's the choices you make that impact your future.

The mindset and beliefs of family members can also influence the behaviors, thus the futures, of those they love.

Well meaning but misinformed loved ones wanting to protect their aging parents may press us to make decisions that impact our futures, almost ensuring we'll decline over time. This is mainly due to health care practitioners' advice; prolific inaccurate articles about aging in magazines, newspapers, and websites; and ignorant mainstream understanding that's been advertised for decades.

If a person hears from their grown children or other family members *don't do this, don't do that, you're too old to do that now, you could fall,* and so on, that person just may stop doing the very things that are helping them to stay functional. They may stop using stairs, taking walks, exercising, mowing the lawn, and so on.

The bold truth is no one ever wants to learn they are wrong. Loved ones really do have their heart in the right place, even if their mindset and understanding may not be. This can be a real problem, so, I want to ask three questions that, when answered honestly, just may provide some revelation for you.

Question #1: *Where Are You?*

I don't mean where do you live or where you are physically.

Where are you in terms of your physical function? Where are you in terms of your health? Where are you in terms of how well or how poorly you're aging?

Have you assessed your diet and lifestyle based on how they impact your risk of experiencing chronic degenerative conditions or chronic pain issues? Other chapters will help with that, if you don't know how. For now, please understand that not knowing where you are now will make it next to impossible to improve your current status and potentially promote decline. I'm thinking you would prefer to maintain your independence when you're in your 90s and beyond. Correct?

Do you plan to age really well, or do you plan to be admitted into a nursing home? Now, I'm not saying anyone ever set a goal of going to a nursing home. I AM saying if you don't set a goal to NOT go there, you just may end up there by default.

Have I got your attention?

Where are you?

To set a course for where you want to go, you need to know your starting point. You need to acknowledge if you're 3,000 miles away from your goal or just 500 feet. Knowing this will allow you to do two things:

1. You'll have a better idea of how much work it'll take to accomplish your goal AND
2. It'll enable you to plan your first step wisely

Let me provide some examples to clear up any confusion.

If you want to be able to easily get on and off the floor, where are you now with that ability?

- Can you get down on the floor without help or do you need to use the sofa for support?
- Are your knees able to bend that much or does pain stop you?
- What about getting back up once down there?
- Do you need something or someone to help pull yourself up?

If you can get down and up without help, how many times do you think you could do that in a row? Was just one try exhausting? Can you do it ten times in a row?

"HELP, I'VE FALLEN AND I CAN'T GET UP!"

Do you remember that commercial? I've worked with people who experienced that very nightmare. One man was on the floor for three days before he was found and hospitalized due to dehydration. He recovered, thank God, but many don't have a good ending to this scenario.

I don't write this to instill fear. I write this to ensure you're honest when you ask yourself the question, "Where am I?" A pie in the sky, head in the sand attitude here can literally leave you in a very bad situation at some point in your life. Knowing where you are now will determine the first steps necessary to enable you to get on and off the floor.

If you can do this without help, but it's tiring after just one rep, you need to do some conditioning to prevent decline. If you need lots of assistance, you may want to seek expert guidance to begin so you don't injure yourself. You wouldn't attempt to begin with a burpee or other squat thrust exercise. But first, you need to know "where are you?"

Don't allow yourself to do nothing about deficits because it's just a normal part of aging. It's NOT normal, just common. Please don't be common!

What about pain?

Do you have a nagging pain that you've been ignoring? Does your back "complain" when you stand up after sitting? Or maybe it aches after cleaning the house or weeding the garden or picking up your grandbaby. You're able to ignore it because it doesn't stop you from doing what needs to get done.

I've worked with many who came to me for help because of shoulder pain, neck pain, knee pain, and so on. When assessed, most admitted they've had back pain off and on over the years but that wasn't important.

That's not why they're here. They're here because of the other pain that's stopping them from doing what needs to get done, making life really hard. It's like they want to sweep the back pain under the rug because they need to "fix" the other reason they're here.

Here's the rub. Typically, the main reason people have more than one area of pain and things get worse is because the initial pain was ignored. Nothing, or very little, was done to address the initial back pain. It didn't stop them and the inconvenience of seeing someone about it outweighed the pain. BUT … the *reason* for that back pain caused a snowball effect into other areas of the body because EVERYTHING IS CONNECTED TO EVERYTHING ELSE.

So, when it comes to pain and physical function, "Where are you?"

Let's look now at health. Do you take multiple prescriptions that cost hundreds of dollars each month? Many do! You may be saying what can I do about that?! I have a heart condition, or I have diabetes. There isn't anything I can do about that. That's not a mindset issue.

Please read Dr. Caldwell Esselstyn's book, *Prevent & Reverse Heart Disease*, OR Dr. Neal Barnard's book, *Program for Reversing Diabetes.* You CAN influence your outcomes with either of these issues quite effectively, and these professionals have the track record to prove it.

There are things you can do, changes you can make, that impact many issues commonly manipulated by medications.

Unfortunately, simply medicating symptoms created by chronic degenerative conditions doesn't prevent the progression of disease, decline, OR serious events from CVD like heart attacks or strokes. Two major factors seen to increase the risk for heart disease are high blood pressure and high cholesterol. Medically manipulating these issues isn't seen in clinical data to prevent death from heart attacks or strokes, as you'll learn soon.

Not being aware of knowledge that can be literally life-altering brings us to the next question I want to ask.

Question #2: *Who Told You ... ?*

Who are you listening to, or, for proper grammar, to whom are you listening?

What source do you trust? Is it:

- your relative or neighbor who just read a best-selling book?
- a YouTube channel that has over 1 million followers?
- a pain management specialist?

The most important question to ask when someone is giving you advice about something as important as your health, physical function, or life is this:

How long have they been doing what they do and how many people have they helped?

I don't mean to step on anyone's toes or sound disrespectful, but just because someone wrote a best-selling book (or two or three) doesn't mean they're actively working with patients. It doesn't mean they can prove what they teach works to eliminate the need for meds or restore function or lengthen lives. It doesn't mean they're wrong either.

The point is to know they can back up what they say with *real-life change.* Not just spout data. The experts I've studied under for decades have helped people eliminate the need for meds, restored pain-free function, and lengthened the lives of those considered to be living on borrowed time for many years. These experts have been doing this for 30 to 40 years or longer. Their track record speaks for itself.

There are some very high-profile researchers with best-selling books and a medical license who are NOT actively practicing medicine. They can't tell you if their research data tranlates into helping real people get better. They can only spout data.

You're not data. I hope you get the idea.

Question #3: *What Are You Doing to Ensure You Age Well?*

Are your actions based on your answer to Question #2?

- Are you taking the latest herb that promises healthy aging?
- Are you counting on medications (ignoring diet and lifestyle) to keep your blood work looking good so your doctor is happy?
- Did you buy that latest ab or other workout device that promises perfect fitness in just three minutes a day?

Many believe memory decline is in large part inevitable because of the effects of biological aging and age-related pathologies. But what if the so-called age-related pathologies really aren't age-related? What if these pathologies are a result of diet and lifestyle choices combined with the time factor? What if the real cause of these things is all about how many years you have NOT been eating well or moving your body?!

This means these issues are *time* related, not *age* related.

Most of the people I've worked with over the last 30 years have heard the following in a medical facility or elsewhere:

- "What do you expect at your age?"
- "Joint pain is a normal part of aging."
- "You shouldn't do that at your age."
- "You're too old to be doing that."

The next time you hear any of these, just reply, "What's age got to do with it?!" *Belief* in popular aging myths and misconceptions is the *real* aging culprit!

The bottom line and real truth?

THERE ARE NO MAGIC PILLS OR SHORTCUTS TO HEALTHY AGING. YOU MUST DO THE WORK.

Want to learn how it happened that my 91-year-old father was not on any meds? Here's what happened.

My mother's voice on the phone was filled with concern. Despite the fact she'd been divorced from my father for years, she called to tell me he was in trouble. His wife had left him. His home required 32 stairs to exit and enter. He was homebound due to his current physical condition. He was also legally blind and hearing impaired.

I visited him immediately and found he had no idea what medications he needed to take or when. There were pill bottles all over the kitchen table and counter. His doctor's office refused to provide any information until they received a notarized document for them to legally provide what I needed. Because there was no time for me to jump through that hoop, I called the homecare office where I worked. They sent a nurse right away to legally get all the necessary medical information by phone and reconcile all my father's medications that day.

Did I mention he was also taking three breathing treatments every day?

Yes, it was a mess alright. When I saw how many meds my dad was taking, I made an appointment with his doctor at the VA. He was amazing! His nickname was Dr. Vish, and he took over 45 minutes with me and my father going over all his meds, many of which he hadn't prescribed. My father had been seeing a lot of different doctors. It was like visiting friends due to his very outgoing social personality. He would always bring a gift when he visited a doctor.

One of the fourteen meds he was taking was for depression. I asked my father if he'd been diagnosed or treated for depression. He answered they put him on that when my brother died. My brother died at age 42 from cancer, nine years prior to that day. My dad was still on the med, and no one had ever tapered or discontinued it in nine years! It's a sad fact they medicated his grief and provided no counseling or therapy, but that's a whole other topic!

With Dr. Vish's oversight, we were able to discontinue all but one of his fourteen medications within just two to three weeks, including the breathing treatments. Those were no longer needed because his ex-wife was a chain smoker, and now that the smoke environment was gone, his breathing was fine.

The last med to go was a blood thinner stopped due to a serious GI bleed requiring emergency surgery. No more blood thinners. No more anything. He was truly medication-free with a restored life of functional strength and independent daily living. He went out daily for lunch with a friend using only a cane for assistance on stairs.

My father had a happy high-quality life for another ten years after stopping all his meds and passed quietly at the age of 93. I firmly believe had he remained on all those meds, he wouldn't have had more than a year or two of very limited existence left.

A prescription pad in the hands of a medical practitioner holds great power. It can save a life. It can also shorten a life due to the compound effects of often-serious side effects. Please don't read what I haven't written. I'm **not** telling you to stop all your meds. I am telling you to ask the all-important question:

"How much will this help me and what are the risks?"

I pray you're now seeing that belief in aging myths and misconceptions is the real culprit behind aging with decline! If improving things with other approaches is known to be beneficial and radically reduces your risk of decline, *why not try them?*

The first step to aging well is to know there's no magic pill that lengthens your life with quality. You can make a marked difference in your future with the right choices.

Next up, are you fully informed?

CHAPTER 2

Meds, Treatments, and Procedures That Are Common After Age 50. Why Ask Why?

MYTH: Medications are necessary.

You just learned the most important question to ask when being advised to take a medication, undergo a procedure, or have surgery:

What are my risks and what are my benefits?

Sounds logical, doesn't it? Are you aware of just how many people don't do this and then regret it later? I have heard the following statement more times than I wish to count in the clinic: *"I wish I knew then what I know now. I wouldn't have agreed to that med ... or procedure ... or surgery."*

This is because the person was still dealing with the fallout months, even years, later. You MUST be informed, which leads to better decisions and improved outcomes.

To ensure you don't miss this information, I'm putting this first as vertigo or dizziness is such a common side effect of many different classes of drugs, including:

- anti-convulsants (often prescribed for pain)
- anti-hypertensives
- antibiotics
- anti-depressants
- anti-psychotics
- anti-inflammatories (NSAIDs)

Please check your med side effects if you suffer from any loss of balance and work with your prescribing practitioner to address this as needed.

It's rare to find an older person who's not on at least two or three medications. Why?

From WebMD[1]: *"As you get older, your doctor is likely to recommend certain medications to improve your health and longevity. These might include a prescription for a specific health concern or over-the-counter remedies like pills, liquids, creams, vitamins, eye drops, or supplements … some health concerns are more common with age, and doctors prescribe medications to help treat them."*

Notice it reads *common* with age, not *normal.* Diseases aren't normal. They're abnormal functioning.

I'm NOT saying anyone should stop taking a prescribed medication without having an informed conversation with their provider.

I AM saying, one more time, *"What's age got to do with it?!"* Sounds like that classic Tina Turner song about love, doesn't it?

Many commonly prescribed treatments and their reported benefits as well as the risks are covered in this chapter. The mostly unknown causes come next. This is what informed decision-making is all about. You aren't required to become a medical expert to make better decisions and experience improved outcomes.

Just become informed of the pros and cons and then decide what's best for you. What risks are you willing to take for what potential benefits that could ensue? Sound logical?

Or you can simply continue to treat symptoms, ignore the causes of what's being medically manipulated, and suffer the side effects of the medical manipulation. Did I mention side effects of commonly prescribed medications require more prescriptions to treat the side effects?

Joyce's story highlights this in a later chapter. Here are the main points:

- *Medication to treat incontinence caused a side effect of tachycardia (rapid heart rate).*
- *Cardiac medication to treat tachycardia caused a side effect of vertigo. Apparently, no one investigated the possibility of sudden onset of tachycardia as a side effect of the incontinence med, despite no cardiac issues found to cause that symptom.*
- *She was prescribed medication to treat the vertigo caused by the cardiac med caused by the incontinence med.*

The absolute worst part? The incontinence medication had no effect. She ended up having bladder suspension surgery and remained on the cardiac and vertigo medications until her death a few years later.

Let's look at four *common* conditions caused by *abnormal* functioning.

Cardiovascular Disease (CVD)

Anti-hypertensive medications: These are given for high blood pressure that injures the circulatory system. These meds are medically logical to prescribe in hopes of preventing a heart attack or a stroke.

How does this play out as far as preventing those things?

What are the risks and benefits of medically manipulating blood pressure? How much does this lower your risk of a heart attack, stroke, or early death and what are the side effects?

A review of 29 studies on the effectiveness and safety of ACE (angiotensin-converting-enzyme) inhibitors showed Lisinopril to be associated with a higher rate of all-cause mortality compared with a placebo.[2]

The kicker reported in this review is *"Some important outcomes such as being readmitted to the hospital and dying from a heart attack were not included because the relevant data were not supplied."* Hmmm …

Conclusion: *"An increase in all-cause mortality combined with a limited effect on reducing systolic and diastolic blood pressure made Lisinopril the worst choice among the ACE inhibitors evaluated."*

In case the thought that other options may be better crosses your mind, the one that did the best was Enalapril, with reported side effects of the highest incidence of cough, kidney failure, and gastrointestinal discomfort.

The SPRINT Trial made headlines recently when researchers reported aggressive medical intervention to get systolic blood pressure below 120 mmHg was so successful at reducing heart disease and strokes it was stopped early so everyone could be treated with this touted to be amazing life-saving strategy. However, the facts don't agree with the headlines.

Although the *relative* risk reduction (playing with the math) showed 26 percent fewer deaths and 38 percent fewer cases of heart failure than those less aggressively medicated, the ACTUAL numbers showed a 0.0117 percent reduction in deaths and 0.0081 percent reduction in heart failure. It pays to have taken graduate level biostatistics courses to understand these studies and how they manipulate the numbers!

Overall, an absolute 0.54 percent reduction in heart attack, heart failure, stroke, and death from heart disease was reported. That's LESS THAN 1 percent in absolute numbers!!!

This underwhelming success came with serious complications such as severe dizziness or fainting, electrolyte imbalances, and kidney damage. Despite these facts the lead researcher stated, *"it seems the benefits outweigh the risks."*

You really can't make this stuff up …

I reported the long list of pain side effects of blood pressure meds in my book, *Pain Culprits!* If you haven't read that book, the most common is chest pain.

Simvastatin: Statin medications are commonly used to treat high cholesterol and fat levels in the blood. They're claimed to reduce the risk of heart attacks, strokes, and other serious medical conditions linked to clogged blood vessels. They're marketed to reduce levels of "bad" cholesterol (LDL) and triglycerides, while increasing levels of "good" cholesterol (HDL).

Let's look at the risks and benefits of medically manipulating cholesterol levels by asking, "How much does this lower your risk of a heart attack, stroke, or early death and what are the side effects?"

According to the evidence, a statin lowers your risk of a heart attack, stroke, or death by less than 3 percent.[3–6] This means great blood work when levels are checked, but you're still at pretty much the same risk of experiencing serious stuff.

I'll never forget a dear, sweet friend of my dad's who was in his 60s. He died from heart failure the day after he was reported to be in perfect health at his doctor's office. His medications were working so well that he had great numbers at his checkup. I'm not writing this to cause fear, but to inform. Medically manipulating blood biomarkers is not the magic pill we've been led to believe.

How about the side effects?

Statins have long been associated with severe muscle weakness. They're also reported to damage skeletal muscle. Side effects include pain, weakness, vomiting, confusion, kidney failure, joint pain, muscle pain, and tendon rupture.[7–9]

I've had patients with muscle pain and weakness when starting these meds have their symptoms dismissed by their physicians. Their concern over the cholesterol levels seems to overshadow the experience of their patients.

If the risks of heart attacks, strokes, or death aren't actually lowered by any appreciable amount, are the side effects worth it? These questions must be asked while having a serious discussion with your prescriber so you can make an informed decision.

Osteoporosis (OP)

Every year, millions of women have a DEXA scan and get diagnosed with osteopenia or osteoporosis.

History of DEXA scans

Before the 1990s, testing for OP was only recommended when a patient presented with fragile bones or unexplainable fractures or breaks. Bone scans were expensive, and community screening wasn't performed. The definition of OP was weakened bones more likely to fracture. It was relatively rare with a very small market for drug treatment.

In 1992, the World Health Organization organized a meeting of experts on bone health to redefine diagnostic and treatment parameters for OP. The new definition was decided as a loss of bone mineral density. This resulted in almost everyone eventually qualifying for a diagnosis because the loss of some bone mineral density is a normal marker for aging. Yes, it's normal to lose some bone density as you age. To be clear, we aren't using the *normal versus common* theme here. It's physiologically normal. This doesn't mean it's a disease that needs to be treated. Let's continue.

An arbitrary level of bone density loss was chosen at this meeting. The panel determined patients who were "borderline" would be labeled as having a new condition called osteopenia, or "pre-osteoporosis."

Merck (pharmaceutical company) was contracted for the development of cheap bone scanning devices to be easily placed in doctors' offices. Merck's marketing department provided leasing programs that made it easier for doctors to have the machines and helped pass a law mandating Medicare to reimburse for the scans.

DEXA stands for dual-energy X-ray absorptiometry. It measures bone density using low-energy X-rays. Because bone blocks a certain amount of X-rays, denser bones equal less X-rays getting through to the detector. A computer then calculates the score.

The T-score rates the amount of bone a person has compared with a young adult of the same gender with peak bone mass. Above −1 is normal. A score between −1 and −2.5 is considered osteopenia and a score below −2.5 is diagnosed as OP. This is claimed to provide an estimate of your risk of fracture. I say "claimed" for a reason. Please read on.

The Z-score rates the amount of bone a person has compared with other people in the same age group and of the same size and gender. If it's unusually high or low, this may indicate a need for further medical tests.

Let's see what the data show regarding the reliability and accuracy of DEXA scans because that's the benchmark for diagnosing and medically treating OP.

Many factors influence the accuracy of DEXA scan results, including:

- machine manufacturer
- technician operating the machine
- patient's clothing
- patient's movement during the scan

The variability can range from 5 to 6 percent. This doesn't seem like much, but changes in bone growth and remodeling are measured down to hundredths or thousandths of a decimal point. A margin of 5 to 6 percent can represent up to ten years of misdiagnosed bone loss!

A New Zealand television show sent a 50-year-old woman to be scanned by two different brands of DEXA machines.[10] One reported she was slightly below normal and the other reported she had OP. Hmmm …

The kicker of all this is loss of bone mineral density is reported to be a *poor predictor* of fracture risk.

Several studies have examined this relationship and reached this conclusion:[11,12] *"We do not recommend a program of screening menopausal women for osteoporosis by measuring bone density."*

The following list of experts currently agree there is insufficient evidence to recommend screening because it doesn't accurately predict future fracture risk:

- Office of Health Technology Assessment, University of British Columbia
- U.S. Preventive Services Task Force
- Swedish Council on Technology Assessment in Health Care
- University of Newcastle Osteoporosis Study Group, Australia
- Effective Health Care Bulletin, United Kingdom

A newer test, Trabecular Bone Scoring (TBS), assesses the actual texture of the bone by looking at the pixel pattern from the DEXA images. It's limited to the lumbar spine at the time of this writing. Because DEXA is designed to only detect bone loss at 30 percent or higher, the TBS is thought to catch what's missed.

The newest testing is the REMS (radiofrequency echo graphic multi-spectrometry). It uses ultrasound to evaluate both bone mineral density and bone quality. Data show it to be 90 percent sensitive but because these are fairly new, there's no data reporting prediction accuracy of a future fracture risk.

Commonly prescribed medications for OP

The following are often prescribed based on the results of a DEXA scan:

- Bisphosphonates
- Parathyroid hormone
- Sclerostin inhibitor

Let's begin with the fact their promoted efficacy has been using relative risk reduction numbers. *Relative* numbers play with math to report a better outcome than what is actually experienced. The *absolute* risk reduction is much lower than what is touted in scientific studies or reported in websites, articles, and magazines. I'll keep it short and sweet as this could easily be an encyclopedia thick (remember those?) tome on this topic.

Bisphosphonates: Brand names include Fosamax, Actonel, Boniva, Aredia, Reclast, and Zometa.

Remember the all-important question. *"How much will this help and what are the risks?"*

The Fracture Intervention Trial showed that after three years, 2.1 percent of women who took Fosamax had fractures, and 3.8 percent of women who took a placebo had fractures.[13]

In *absolute* terms this is a 1.7 percent risk reduction, but it's reported as a 44 percent reduction in *relative* terms:

- REAL math: 3.8 – 2.1 = 1.7 percent.
- RELATIVE math: 2.1 is 44 percent of 3.8.

This is how they ensure an intervention sounds like it works better than it does.

What about the risks?

You must remain upright for at least 30 minutes after taking bisphosphonate as it can cause serious injury to the esophagus.

My mom had severe pain after taking this med and rushed to the ER thinking she was having a heart attack. They found a burn injury to her esophagus from the medication. You can imagine her horror upon learning this since she'd lost her 42-year-old son (my brother) to esophageal cancer.

All bisphosphonates slow bone resorption by blocking the action of osteoclasts, which resorb older, weakened bone. Osteoblasts then lay down new bone. The problem is osteoblast activity is stimulated by osteoclast activity so medically manipulating this process leads to bone fragility and an increased risk of fracture.

Say what?!

Yes, the very reason the drug is prescribed is to "prevent" fractures, yet it's seen to decrease bone strength in the data:

"Fosomax significantly suppresses bone remodeling and increases microdamage accumulation, leading to a decline in bone strength of 20% for patients taking the drug compared to placebo."[14]

Dr. Dean Lorich reported 20 cases in which a fracture sheared the thigh bone with little or no trauma. Of those 20 patients, 19 had been taking Fosamax for an average of 6.9 years.[15] *"The risk of atypical fracture among women increased progressively with the duration of use ..."*

Other studies confirm atypical femoral fractures with use of this med.[16]

Dental records of 13,000 patients at the University of Southern California's dental school clinic showed 4 percent of patients taking Fosamax had osteonecrosis of the jaw.[17]

Osteo (bone) necrosis (cell death) is seen in the jaw bones of patients taking these drugs so it's a real concern to dentists when providing care.

Let's look at the other meds to see if they're any less risky and if they provide more benefit than 1.7 percent fracture risk reduction.

Parathyroid hormones: Brand names include Forteo and Tymlos.

Parathyroid hormones (PTH) regulate how much calcium in the diet:

- body absorbs
- bones store
- kidneys secrete

These medications are an artificial form of PTH reported to increase bone mineral density and strength and reduce fracture risk. Do they?

A study that looked at risk reduction of new vertebral and nonvertebral fractures over 18 months compared Forteo, Tymlos, and placebo.[18]

New spine fracture rates were reported as follows:

- Foteo: 0.73 percent
- Tymlos: 0.48 percent
- Placebo: 3.65 percent

Yes, these numbers show a difference, but the absolute math is a reduction risk of new spine fracture being only 2.92 percent for Forteo and 3.17 percent for Tymlos. Researchers also reported that the study wasn't large enough to determine if the drug really reduced the risk of fractures.

Do the risks outweigh the benefits? The FDA requires a warning label as a risk of bone cancer is seen in animal studies.[19] This is why insurance companies only pay for two years of treatment and then bisphosphonates are prescribed for lifelong "maintenance." So, these newer classes of drugs don't even eliminate the need for prescribing bisphosphonates.

Pain is experienced in over 20 percent of those taking the drug. Other side effects include low or high blood pressure, palpitations, chest pain, nausea, vomiting, hiatus hernia, gastro-esophageal reflux disease, constipation, diarrhea, dyspepsia, gastrointestinal disorder, tooth disorder, depression, insomnia, vertigo, fatigue, asthenia, and syncope.

Details provided on the Tymlos site include the following:

"Some people may feel dizzy, have a faster heartbeat, or feel lightheaded soon after the TYMLOS injection is given … If your symptoms get worse or do not go away, stop taking TYMLOS and call your healthcare provider."

"TYMLOS can cause some people to have a higher blood calcium level than normal … Tell your healthcare provider if you have nausea, vomiting, constipation, low energy, or muscle weakness ..."

"TYMLOS can cause some people to have higher levels of calcium in their urine than normal. Increased calcium may also cause you to develop kidney stones (urolithiasis) in your kidneys, bladder, or urinary tract ..."

So once again, I ask:

Do the benefits outweigh the risks?

Sclerostin inhibitor: Brand name Evenity.

The treatment benefits show a 0.5 percent occurrence of new spine fractures in the treatment group, and a 1.8 percent occurrence of new spine fractures in the placebo group.[20] That's an *absolute* risk reduction of 1.3 percent. The *relative* risk reduction? 73 percent.

Clinical fracture risk reduction reported at 12 months isn't as impressive, even in relative terms. It's only 36 percent but 0.9 percent in absolute terms.

The numbers improve if you're looking at the 24-month mark for reported nonvertebral fractures. *Relative* risk reduction is 75 percent. *Absolute* risk reduction is 1.9 percent.

Side effects include joint pain, muscle spasms, neck pain, osteonecrosis of the jaw, atypical femoral fracture, peripheral edema, headache, insomnia, and anti-drug antibodies. It's also reported to increase a woman's risk of having a heart attack and stroke, with a boxed warning to not be prescribed to women with other cardiovascular risk factors.

I think you're getting the idea there are many risks with these medications. Now you can decide if the benefits outweigh the risks by having an informed conversation with your prescribing practitioner.

Please be sure to read the other chapters so you can learn about bone strength and what you can do to safely reduce your risk of fractures no matter your age.

Osteoarthritis (OA)

This topic is big, but I'll do my best to provide important facts that aren't well known but should be in the rest of this chapter.

Common treatments for OA include pain medications, anti-inflammatories, corticosteroid injections, and surgeries.

Now for *"How much will this help me and what are my risks?"*

Medications for OA

A review of 15 studies with over 6,000 participants showed that acetaminophen was found to reduce hip or knee pain better than placebo by 4 points on a scale of 0–100.[21] In plain English, this means if you scored your pain at 50/100, it'll be reduced to 46/100. Kinda useless, or is it just me?

The topper is that physical function and stiffness were considered about the same between the medication and the placebo. It wouldn't be so bad if there weren't some serious side effects such as acute liver failure, liver transplant, or death.[22]

My dad, who became medicated the last two months of his life, literally turned yellow just two days before he died as the acetaminophen he was given for joint pain overtaxed his liver. He was 93. The fact is that many people are already overtaxing their livers due to health issues and other meds. So, a simple over-the-counter pain reliever can be the tipping point. You must know this fact.

Moving on to anti-inflammatory meds.

Non-steroidal anti-inflammatory drugs (NSAIDs) were reviewed by the *British Medical Journal*.[23] They reviewed 23 studies with over 10,000 participants and how effective NSAIDs were for symptomatic OA of the knee.

Are you ready for a fact most people have never heard of? Clinical studies have what's called inclusion and exclusion criteria. This means they pick and choose the subjects approved into the study. Thirteen of the studies reviewed in this report excluded participants from the study if they didn't respond to NSAIDs. Can you say *stacking the deck in your favor*?

Of the twenty-three trials, sixteen were sponsored by the pharmaceutical industry and three reported the address of a pharmaceutical company as the workplace of most of the authors. This means only four had a lower risk of bias.

Despite this bias (and stacking the deck), the overall difference, short term, was reported to be 15.6 percent better for NSAIDs than placebo after two to thirteen weeks. Only one trial looked at long-term effect (one to four years) and no significant effect of NSAIDs was seen when compared with a placebo.

The conclusion?

"NSAIDs can reduce short term pain in osteoarthritis of the knee slightly better than placebo, but the current analysis does not support long term use of NSAIDs for this condition. As serious adverse effects are associated with oral NSAIDs, only limited use can be recommended."

NSAID risks are numerous and prevalent. There are currently over 22,000 published studies.[24–26] Use is linked to GI-bleeding-related deaths and increased risk of serious cardiac issues. Long-term use is associated with stomach irritation, ulcers, heartburn, diarrhea, fluid retention, kidney dysfunction, and cardiovascular disease.

I have a close family member who was taking NSAIDs regularly for joint pain. Her stomach became a literal mess and when she stopped the meds, she found her pain didn't increase. Other actions she'd taken had improved her joint function without knowing it and she mistakenly thought the med was decreasing her pain. It wasn't.

Another fact you must know, especially if you care about muscle health and strength as you age. NSAIDs have been seen to inhibit muscle growth when performing resistance training to quadriceps.[27]

Let's look now at steroid injections. I'm staying on OA of the knee to keep this from becoming overwhelming data, yet please know similar or worse reports are seen for OA of other areas such as the hip.

A 2017 study showed patients with symptomatic knee OA who received two years of intra-articular triamcinolone compared with intra-articular saline resulted in significantly greater cartilage volume loss and no significant difference in knee pain.[28]

"These findings do not support this treatment for patients with symptomatic knee osteoarthritis" was the published conclusion.

What about the risks listed by the manufacturer?[29] They include the following:

- death of nearby bone (osteonecrosis)
- joint infection
- nerve damage
- deterioration of cartilage

- tendon weakening or rupture
- thinning of nearby bone (osteoporosis)

I mentioned the FDA black box warning on corticosteroids regarding spinal injections in my book, *Pain Culprits!* There are severe and serious risks when injected into the epidural space of the spine, including "loss of vision, stroke, paralysis, and death."[30]

The last stop for this topic is regarding surgeries and imaging. You may wonder why on Earth I would talk about imaging because that's not a treatment. Treatments are often based on image reports. What if image reports aren't an accurate picture of why you have joint pain?

Many studies have shown that symptoms and imaging results don't line up, meaning the pain may not be caused by what shows on the X-ray or MRI. It's reported that *"radiographic (X-ray) knee osteoarthritis is an imprecise guide to the likelihood that knee pain or disability will be present … The results of knee X-rays should not be used in isolation when assessing individual patients with knee pain."*[31]

In the U.S., knee replacements are expected to increase by 400 percent in the next 16 years![32] This is nearly 3.5 MILLION projected surgeries! Hip replacements are expected to increase by 284 percent!

Given that the cause of joint damage, reported in the next chapter, has been found, why aren't these surgeries decreasing in number?

In 2019, Germany, Switzerland, Austria, Finland, and Belgium were among the countries with the highest rates for hip and knee replacement. This is truly a worldwide problem.

Although joint replacements can be a real need for those with severe joint damage and pain, wouldn't it be nice to prevent such a thing from being necessary in the first place?

I've worked with people who've been able to restore function without surgery by doing the right things the right way. Have you exhausted all options? It may not be too late to try.

Surgeries intended to "clean up" the arthritic joint have been shown to be a colossal waste of time and resources. There's no evidence the arthritis is cured or arrested by arthroscopic surgery. In older uncontrolled studies (no control group), about half reported pain relief, yet the physiological basis for the pain relief remains unclear.

A controlled study comparing lavage, debridement, and placebo had a surprising conclusion.[33] The placebo group did NOT have surgery and they did just as well with pain relief and improvement in function as the other two groups that DID have surgery.

A recent review of 16 *controlled* studies concluded:[34] *"Arthroscopic surgery provides little or no clinically important benefit in pain or function, probably does not provide clinically important benefits in knee-specific quality of life, and may not improve treatment success compared with a placebo procedure ..."*

Urinary Incontinence (UI)

What about all the medical intervention provided to those who seek help for unwanted leakage?

Does it work? What are the risks?

You may be one who had a good outcome different from what is written next, yet for many, the fallout of making uninformed decisions can be devastating.

The purpose of being informed is to make the right decision for you based on facts. If you feel certain benefits outweigh the risks, your decision was not made in ignorance.

Common incontinence recommendations include the following:

- Spacing fluid intake and limiting fluids before bedtime
- Limiting alcohol and caffeine intake
- Bladder training
- Kegel exercises
- Medications
- Surgery

If simply following the recommendations to space fluid intake and limiting fluids before bedtime worked, the countless options for adult diapers would not be available. This strategy is more about not getting up in the middle of the night, rushing to the toilet, and risking a fall.

Considering the high intake of both caffeine and alcohol in our world, I believe everyone would be incontinent if this was the actual CAUSE of the issue. I've worked with folks who developed the ability to drink coffee and go for a run without fear of leakage.

Yes, these substances inhibit your antidiuretic hormone, so they sort of trick your body into losing fluid. They basically work as diuretics, but I see this as *exposing an existing issue* if UI occurs when drinking either caffeine or alcohol. They don't cause the problem; they simply expose it.

What about bladder training? I've seen this used often in nursing home settings. My heart always went out to the resident, suffering from dementia, who kept asking to go to the bathroom but was told they needed to wait until it was time because they were "training" their bladder. REALLY?! Making someone wait does NOT strengthen their pelvic floor.

The bladder can only hold as much urine without leaking as the pelvic floor muscles can support. Often, these poor folks would end up wetting themselves and then need to be cleaned and changed.

Looking at studies that support bladder training as an effective strategy, the *efficacy* is less than impressive. One well done prospective study showed frequency, nighttime need to urinate, and urgency all improved, yet the improvement of *actual incontinence* was not significant.[35] This study was done on a younger population with an average age of 57 years, not dementia patients in a nursing home setting.

Yes, bladder training may show some small, specific benefits for certain populations in a study or two; however, there are a lot of variables to consider. It's truly restricted to those who are physically and cognitively able and motivated with full comprehension.

A large review of 15 trials and over 2,000 subjects reported the following conclusion in 2023 about bladder training:[36] *"Most of the evidence was low or very-low certainty … There may be no difference in efficacy or safety between bladder training and PFMT (pelvic floor muscle training). More well-designed trials are needed to reach a firm conclusion."*

As you saw, low or very low certainty is not something that instills confidence in the outcome.

Kegel exercises are presented in chapter 5 in detail as that entire chapter is dedicated to UI.

Medications for UI

Anticholinergics are prescribed to treat an overactive bladder requiring up to 12 weeks to take effect. My question is what's causing the bladder to abnormally contract?

Side effects include the following:

- heartburn
- blurry vision
- rapid heartbeat (tachycardia)
- flushed skin
- urinary retention
- impaired memory and confusion

Efficacy

A 2021 study[37] reported risk to the elderly due to the cognitive side effects. The number of new agents, including botulism A, for pharmacological treatment of UI reported in depth was staggering. Yes, a reduction in bladder contractions was reported as well as voiding frequency but ...

The International Consultation on Incontinence Research Society (ICI-RS) stressed the need for new research exploring OAB (overactive bladder) phenotyping through urodynamics, functional brain imaging, and psychology.

There's a lot of potential harm seen with these drugs. They have a long way to go to reach more benefit than potential harm. The high target population being nursing home or homebound people with cognitive deficits makes this a serious concern.

Other medications include:

- Myrbetriq to relax the bladder muscle so it will hold more urine. Side effects include nausea, diarrhea, constipation, dizziness, headache, and increased blood pressure.

- Tofranil (a tricyclic antidepressant) used to treat combination urge and stress UI. Side effects include irregular heartbeat, low blood pressure with a risk of fainting, dry mouth, blurry vision, and constipation. I'm not including the psychiatric side effects, which you may want to research because they're quite staggering.
- Cymbalta (SNRI) to help the sphincter relax. Side effects include nausea, dry mouth, dizziness, constipation, insomnia, and fatigue. Not to be taken with chronic liver disease. Also with some serious psychiatric side effects …
- Topical estrogen to "rejuvenate" the tissues. Not to be used if there is a history of breast cancer or uterine cancer.

Surgeries

I believe society will eventually see the surgeries performed for this issue as barbaric as the ancient use of leaches, bloodletting, and arsenic in the emerging field of medicine. Shocked? Just read on …

Surgeries for men include:

- Male sling placed around the end of the urethra to compress it and prevent leaking involves making a cut between the scrotum and anus. Risks: urine retention requiring a second surgery, bleeding, infection (mesh, bone area, and pubic bone), and erosion with recurrent leakage.
- Implanted artificial sphincter using a cuff to close the urethra. Squeezing the pump releases urine when needed. Risks: pain, bleeding, infection, injury to urethra, surgery to remove or replace it, ongoing leakage, permanent problems urinating, and catheterization.
- A pacemaker-like device stimulating nerves to relax the bladder and pelvic floor muscles. Surgically implanted under the skin close to the tailbone. Risks: pain, infection, wire movement, changes in bowel or urinary function, and unpleasant feeling of stimulation.

Surgeries for women include:

- Vaginal sling placed around the neck of the bladder to support it and prevent leaking, requiring a cut in the abdomen and vagina. Complications can occur even many years later. Risks: bladder perforation, erosion of the mesh into the vagina and painful intercourse, infection, urinary problems, recurrent incontinence, bleeding, vaginal scarring, and neuromuscular problems.
- Colposuspension involves making a cut in your abdomen, lifting the neck of your bladder, and stitching it in this lifted position. Risks: difficulty emptying the bladder completely, chronic UTIs, and painful intercourse.
- Augmentation cystoplasty involves making your bladder bigger by adding a piece of tissue from your intestine into the bladder wall. Risks: may need to use a catheter to empty the bladder and chronic urinary tract infections.
- Urinary diversion whereby the tubes from your kidneys to your bladder are redirected outside the body to collect urine in a bag. Risks: bladder infection and more surgery due to complications.
- Urethral bulking agents injected to increase the size of the urethral walls, allowing the urethra to stay closed with more force. Risks: less effective and often needs to be repeated.

There are other treatments that include sacral nerve stimulation and posterior tibial nerve stimulation. Efficacy is reportedly sketchy for these.

In conclusion, there are many safe, and often very effective, strategies you can apply in your own life provided later in this book.

All medical treatment carries risks. There is no magic pill that fixes anything without any side effects or potential harm. Asking the all-important question *"how much will this help and what are my risks?"* is key to making better decisions with improved outcomes.

You must weigh your risks and benefits.

CHAPTER 3

Known and Unknown Causes, Oh No! What Can You Do About It?

MYTH: Aging well is pure luck.

"People will think *I'm stupid!" I was taken aback as my 102-year-old patient, lying in a hospital bed, said this to me. She'd had a mild bout of pneumonia and needed to recover her strength after lying in bed for three days. Her goal was to return to a living environment that required her to be independent in the daily tasks of life. If she didn't recover her previous function, she would be looking at nursing home placement.*

I'll share the reason she said that later. First, I want to report some not so well known facts about what's reported to be the cause(s) of some very important issues.

I agree wholeheartedly with Dr. Joel Robbins, MD, DC, who said: *"The smarter we get, the sicker we become, because we are looking for cures instead of causes."*

Let's begin with the real cause behind cardiovascular disease.

Cardiovascular Disease (CVD)

CVD ends lives much earlier than they should end. I write the following not to instill fear but to inform. The first sign of heart disease 40 percent of the time is sudden death. Plus, 50 percent of those who die from a heart attack were told by their doctor their health was okay six months prior to the event.

To be blunt, if you're medically manipulating blood biomarkers and told your bloodwork looks great, the underlying REASON for CVD is NOT resolved by medications. The symptoms improve. The bloodwork improves. The last chapter informed you the risk of events happening are only slightly reduced: a less than 3 percent reduction in risk for a heart attack, stroke, or death.

I'll never forget arriving at a family member's home and watching him being loaded into the ambulance after getting a panicked call from his daughter. He died on the way to the hospital. He was 44 years old with no known history of CVD.

The brother of my mom's best friend died suddenly of a heart attack just one day after being told he was in good health. All his bloodwork looked good. He was told to keep taking his meds to manipulate his blood pressure, cholesterol, and more. He died at the age of 47 with great bloodwork.

Let's look at why this happens.

Human physiology and healthy blood circulation

Your blood vessels are lined with endothelial cells, which are a powerhouse of production and activity. They do the following pretty much 24/7:

- Feed every cell and organ via blood supply
- Regulate blood flow and blood pressure
- Regulate the size of your arteries
- Resist injury by bacteria, viruses, toxins, and pollution
- Manufacture hormones and chemical messengers
- Balance inflammation/anti-inflammation system
- Balance clotting systems and platelets

As you can see, these are very busy cells. So, what happens if they become injured? Endothelial dysfunction.

Endothelial cells produce nitric oxide (NO), keeping blood vessels open wide to prevent the constriction that increases blood pressure, the buildup of plaques, and the risk of clots that lead to strokes and heart attacks. It would seem prudent to protect them from damage, don't you think?

Did you know erectile dysfunction (ED) meds work by increasing the production of nitric oxide? When I attended a conference in 2015, one of the expert speakers, a cardiovascular surgeon, presented *Erectile Dysfunction, The Canary in the Coal Mine.*

If someone is experiencing ED, they have CVD. It just hasn't been diagnosed yet. Aging *well* doesn't include problems with intimacy, does it?

So, what causes damage to these precious, hard-working cells?

- High blood pressure (increases as cell damage increases)
- Insulin resistance (impacts NO production)[1]
- Glycation (due to a unique relationship with glucose)[2]
- Inflammation (pro-inflammatory mediators lead to endothelial cell death)[3]
- Oxidative stress (promotes endothelial dysfunction)[4]
- Toxins (high cholesterol, high blood sugar, smoking, inflammation)[5]

As you can see, nothing on this list points to genetics. Hmmm ...

Let's see what food has to do with the above, shall we?

There are countless studies that connect diet with high blood pressure. Foods reported to "treat" high blood pressure or help prevent it are vegetables, fruits, legumes, and whole grains. A focus on the diet being no more than 15 percent total fat and limiting animal foods to 10 percent of total food intake is also critical. This means high-fat foods and foods loaded with cholesterol are not your friend if you wish to protect your endothelial cells.

Unfortunately, when you read mainstream websites, there's a lot of inaccurate information regarding what constitutes a diet that protects circulation. For instance, the DASH diet (listed on the Mayo Clinic site) tells you to focus on plant foods but also states animal foods can be consumed up to six times a day. Yes, they're 1-ounce servings or one egg. Who eats just 1 ounce of chicken, and can you really consume up to six eggs a day and prevent CVD? REALLY?!!!

They also tell you it's fine to consume up to three servings of fats and oils per day and up to three 1.5-ounce servings a day of low-fat cheese. However, 1.5 ounces of the average "low fat" cheese contains 9 grams of fat, which is 81 calories of pure fat in a 135-calorie serving. How is something 60 percent fat considered low-fat?!

Did you know cheese is labeled low fat simply because it's less fat than the original? There is NO SUCH THING as low-fat cheese … not to mention the cholesterol and estrogen contained within. Yes, estrogen.

Other sites that promote the DASH diet are WebMD, Heart.org, and NIH.gov. It gets even more confusing when you look at the list of foods promoted as heart healthy, reportedly going through a rigorous process to be included. Here are just a few foods reported as heart healthy. The fat and cholesterol in a 4-ounce serving is provided:

- Ground beef 96 percent lean (~28 percent fat and 65 mg cholesterol)
- Pork tenderloin (~37 percent fat and 74 mg cholesterol)
- Pork sirloin (~37 percent fat and 95 mg cholesterol)
- Boneless, skinless chicken breasts (~20 percent fat and 86 mg cholesterol)

I'm hoping you see that although chicken has less fat when you remove the skin, the cholesterol is basically the same as all the others. I'm NOT telling you not to eat chicken. I'm simply providing facts of which you may not have been aware. Chicken is not really a healthy food because all animal foods have cholesterol and saturated fat, which can harm your endothelial cells.

Limiting animal food intake to 10 percent of your total intake means eating plant foods for most of your meals and including animal foods (optional, not necessary) just two to three times per week. This is shown in the data to radically reduce your risk of developing CVD and a whole lot of other nasty diseases that no one wants. Please read *The China Study* by T. Colin Campbell, Ph.D.

Taking the risk to continue swimming against the current of mainstream knowledge, I want to inform you it's a fact that ALL oils are seen to damage endothelial cells. Many studies have shown monounsaturated fat (olive oil) can progress artery disease as much as saturated fat.[6]

Endothelial dysfunction is seen when olive oil is consumed. Both omega-3 and omega-6 are reported to contribute to the development of plaques, damaging the arteries.[7–9]

Taking omega-3 was NOT seen to reduce the risk of heart attacks, strokes, or death according to a review of 89 published studies.[10]

This means there's no magic pill that protects your circulation. Food and movement are the only real answers to aging well. Please read Dr. Caldwell Esselstyn's book, *Prevent & Reverse Heart Disease*. He's provided education to his patients for decades that has enabled them to live healthy lives long after serious cardiac issues occurred. All with simple dietary changes.

Degenerative Disc Disease (DDD)

Dr. Leena Kauppila, a brilliant research expert, has published extensive studies on the relationship between impaired lumbar circulation and DDD. I was exposed to her work at a conference many years ago. The title of her talk was *Back Pain and Disc Degeneration as Manifestations of Cardiovascular Disease*. I booked a flight just to hear her presentation.

Dr. Kauppila has thoroughly studied the arteries of the lumbar spine and their relationship to low-back health. She reports a prevalent association of impaired artery circulation with low back pain, degenerative disc disease, disc herniations, spinal stenosis, and more.

Here are the highlights of her studies.

Lumbar arteries and what they supply:

1. Posterior Body Wall: muscles around your spine, etc.
2. Vertebral Body and Nerve Root: vertebrae, nerve roots, etc.
3. Posterior Peritoneum: psoas and quadratum lumborum (deep hip muscles)

What's seen with impaired circulation:

1. Pain related to exercise and accumulation of lactic acid and muscle atrophy.
2. Dull, constant pain, end-plate sclerosis, disc degeneration, sciatica, and others.
3. Lateral back pain and pain with hip muscle activity.

This is very real, factual data that underlines the importance of your circulatory health when it comes to chronic back pain, DDD, and more. Aging *well* does not coexist with these issues, does it?

Atherosclerosis and disc degeneration are seen to coincide, meaning those that have CVD are also seen to have DDD. This was observed in the Framingham Study and the Nurses' Health Study. These studies are HUGE, with massive numbers of subjects and decades of follow-up.

In Dr. Kauppila's direct studies, she noted DDD was associated with impaired lumbar and middle sacral arteries. She also noted that patients with above-normal LDL cholesterol had more severe neurogenic symptoms, more severe back pain, and occluded arteries more often.[11] Sciatica was also strongly and consistently associated with impaired lumbar blood supply.

Other researchers have seen an association between sciatica and high cholesterol levels. Smoking (no surprise here) is also associated with an increase in low back pain, DDD, and disc herniation.[12–15]

Thankfully, there are things you can do to improve this. Specifically, exercise and diet. Exercise helps create collateral arteries that bypass impaired arteries to provide blood supply. It's called angiogenesis. Your body literally births new blood vessels when stimulated properly with movement. Yes, angiogenesis can be detrimental if cancer cells are releasing chemicals to stimulate their own blood supply, yet that's a topic not addressed in this book. I will state food impacts this aspect of angiogenesis in a very beneficial way, so please eat your veggies!

Fruits and veggies are so powerful, they help with angiogenesis in addition to protecting those precious endothelial cells mentioned previously. This means a low-fat, whole-food, plant-based way of eating not only helps with CVD but also with DDD and a host of painful ailments no one wants in their life if they desire to age well.

Osteoporosis (OP)

Please remember, it isn't a simple, logical deduction that low bone density equals fracture, as you learned in the last chapter. Because DEXA scans measure the amount of minerals in the bones and not their strength to resist fracture, let's look at why or how mineral content of bone decreases.

Given that the female body stores more minerals in her childbearing years to provide for a growing fetus and producing breast milk for two years after delivery, a bone mineral density (BMD) test shows a high mineral content at this age. After childbearing years, the body releases nearly 2 pounds of minerals because they're no longer needed. Now, a BMD test reports a deficiency, which isn't really logical when human physiology is understood.

Thankfully, mineral content doesn't directly correlate to bone strength OR fracture rates, which depends on other dense connective tissues, not just minerals. There are other factors that play a pivotal role in bone strength. Surprised?

That stated, let's look at what has the potential to weaken bones so they're at a higher risk of fracture AND what can be done effectively to prevent it or potentially reverse it. Because there certainly are people with very weak and fragile bones who've experienced fractures, it behooves us to research the cause behind it.

There's a great deal of scientific evidence showing a high intake of acid food is associated with the need for the bones' stored buffering agents (carbonates, citrates, and other alkaline materials) to neutralize the acid load.[16] This means minerals in bone are used as a tool for homeostasis, which is a self-regulating process your body uses to maintain life.

The pH of your blood needs to remain between 7.35 and 7.45 to maintain life. This delicate balance requires protection from the high acid load of animal foods, which include meat, poultry, fish, eggs, dairy, and cheese. There has been some recent data disputing this fact, yet "calcium-in and calcium-out" has been the subject of nearly countless research studies for many decades. If more calcium goes out of the body than comes in, this leaves a negative balance. Chapter 9 provides more detail about low-acid eating, so let's look at another factor here.

Mineral content is not the only thing that provides real strength to our bones so, what else does?

Bone strength

Bone strength specifically refers to the bone's ability to withstand force prior to fracture. It's physiologically linked with fatigue resistance to repetitive loads.[17] Your bones are amazing! They're highly adaptive, structurally dynamic, and metabolically active. They're superior to all other body structures in terms of strength and toughness. Wow!

Your bones rely on and respond to the physiological and mechanical demands placed upon them. This means not only do they provide buffering agents when needed, they also respond to mechanical loads that occur consistently by increasing in toughness. Translation? Being sedentary weakens bones.

There's another issue you must know about in case this is relevant to you. Your endocrine system mediates a complex process of calcium-phosphate balance, energy metabolism, and bone mineralization in response to ever-changing physiological needs.

In plain English, your endocrine function plays a major role in bone health, especially as you age. If hormonal imbalances and environmental irregularities exist, endocrine function can become deficient at preserving healthy bone structure.

This is the reason the latest class of medications was developed to target parathyroid hormone function. You read the risks and benefits with those drugs in the last chapter.

To conclude this section in simple terms, the most important strategies for healthy bones are diet and movement. Low-acid eating is important. This doesn't mean not eating citrus foods. They don't cause an acid load upon digestion. They're actually alkaline in that process. Cool, huh?

It's not the pH of the food *before* digestion. It's what happens *afterward* that counts.

The movement strategy means you want to be performing safe, weight-bearing resistance exercises for healthy bones as long as you are above ground. Please read Part 3 for more details and check the Resources if you don't know where to start.

Osteoarthritis (OA)

Simply stated, the most unknown cause of joint *damage* is chronic inflammation in the body, and diet is well known to influence inflammation.

The most unknown cause of joint *pain* is poor joint biomechanics. Being sedentary or training inauthentically can lead to pain, stiffness, and injury.

Chronic inflammation

Reasons a person may be in a chronic inflammatory state include:

1. High intake of animal foods (anything with a face or a mother, even if it swims)
2. Excess body weight
3. Lack of or low intake of whole grains, cruciferous vegetables, and fiber

Animal foods contain arachidonic acid (AA). This is an essential fatty acid, which means we must get it from food; however, your body converts the healthy fats in plant foods (linoleic acid) to AA. This means you don't need to get it directly from animal foods, which includes dairy. Yes, dairy is an animal food.

When you consume animal foods every day at every meal, your body over-responds during the normal healing and repair process. An oversupply of AA is like putting a brick on the gas pedal, promoting chronic inflammation in your body.

The USDA's Standard 13 and 16 databases report animal proteins produce the highest amounts of AA in the body. Fruits, vegetables, grains, and legumes (beans/lentils) produce little or no AA. Processed baked goods produce a moderate amount.

Another source of chronic inflammation is excess body weight. Fat cells produce inflammatory cytokines, which are proteins that serve as messengers between cells. They bind to target immune cells, triggering an excessive immune response that can lead to inflammation and tissue destruction.

Some good news about this is that I have seen many people experience less pain rather quickly by changing their diet even BEFORE they've had enough time to lose weight. Of course, losing excess weight is important, but I didn't want you to think you'd be stuck in pain until that can be achieved. Changing what you put in your mouth can have a profound effect on your symptoms in as little as one week!

Another potential reason for joint pain that has nothing to do with diet is impaired joint biomechanics. Your body works as a whole, not just as a sum of its parts. This means pain in one joint is often due to impaired function in another area. The thing is, it's not always because of OA!

Because impaired biomechanics isn't a chronic degenerative condition, it's covered in detail later. The good news is you can do something about it!

Hopefully, you've seen just how much of what mainstream understanding is missing details that matter. You can only do the right things if you know what those right things to do are. If you think you're doing a good thing for your health by removing the skin from the chicken and eliminating carbs, the lack of success those things achieve will lead you to believe there's nothing you can do.

That couldn't be further from the truth. As you just read, there are LOTS of things you can do that breed success.

CHAPTER 4

Nursing Home Placement Is a Goal No One Set, Ever

MYTH: Aging means loss of independence.

I'll always remember *my first encounter with Sue. Her family was concerned because she was having a lot of chronic pain issues that impacted her ability to do all she wanted to do.*

As I assessed her function, how mobile her joints were, and how stabile her movement was, I realized decline was imminent for her if something didn't change soon. The sad part of this story is the fact Sue was regularly seeing multiple professionals to treat her problems. She was seeing a chiropractor every week, an acupuncturist, a physical therapist, and a massage therapist less often but still frequently. When I asked her about her exercise program she stated, "I hate exercise and have never done it. I'm busy enough with housework."

Because assessments require me to report honestly, it was necessary for me to tell Sue my professional opinion. If she didn't start actively working to restore strength and balance, she would likely need a walker in less than five years. You may be surprised to hear what Sue thought of me during that encounter, which she admitted a couple of months later.

I'll share what Sue had to say after I cover the facts about why loss of independence REALLY happens. Spoiler alert. The facts have little to do with age and THERE IS NO MAGIC PILL.

Yes, we see people in their "golden years" using all kinds of devices to help them get from point A to point B. We see the use of canes, walkers, and wheelchairs by many of the elderly population. BUT we also see many in their 80s and beyond NOT using these devices, even running marathons!

So, what happens to some and not to others? Why do so many decline, lose their independence, and end up in a nursing home? Given that *no one ever sets a goal to go to a nursing home,* why do so many end up there?

The short answer is they were most likely sedentary and did little exercise as they aged. Yes, I'm well aware there are those who have serious medical conditions or severe pain that hinders active exercise. I'm not speaking of those situations. I'm speaking of those I've met so often, like Sue, who say, *"Oh, I never liked exercise."* This was spoken almost always as they looked up at me from their chair with a walker perched in front of them.

I'm not judging anyone and I mean no disrespect. I'm simply pointing out what I've seen and heard for the last 30 years. The majority of those who declined were those who led mostly sedentary lives. They expressed dislike of exercise and were quite reluctant to do any movement with me during a therapy session. It was a total disconnect between their current lack of physical function and their attitude toward conditioning their body. I also saw a huge difference in the foods present on their kitchen counters, but that's another chapter.

Sarcopenia

Sarcopenia is a Greek term meaning "poverty of flesh." It's used to describe the decrease in lean body mass (muscle) commonly seen with aging. Countless sources report that around the age of 45, muscle mass begins to decline at a rate of ~1 percent per year with increasing body fat mass.

Here's the spoiler alert. It's not due to aging. This gradual loss of muscle has clearly been tied to lack of exercise.

I recently did a deep dive into the data while preparing for a Power Aging Boot Camp event. Sarcopenia is commonly defined *as age-related lean muscle loss;* however, I modified this definition after my research was done. I'll share that shortly.

The thing about sarcopenia is that although a person may see little change in their size over the decades, their body composition will be a much unhealthier ratio of fat to lean muscle. When you look at a picture of sarcopenia (found easily with an internet search), the composition between a younger person and an INACTIVE 60-year-old will show a big difference in amount of muscle and fat. Notice the capital letters? More on that is coming up.

There'll be more fat tissue and less muscle mass seen with sarcopenia. This will be the person who has trouble with the physical tasks of daily life, like squatting, lifting, or getting down on the floor and back up without assistance. They'll need help getting out of the car or off a low toilet. This is someone plopping when they sit. They're declining and, if nothing is done to reverse this, they'll often end up in a nursing home.

Did you know physical inactivity is reported by the World Health Organization as the fourth leading risk factor for death globally? It comes after high blood pressure, tobacco use, and high blood sugar. It is reported that 6 percent of deaths across the globe, an estimated 3.2 million preventable deaths each year, result from physical inactivity. People are literally dying *before their time* because they weren't active.

Here's a partial list of the consequences of sarcopenia:

- Increased risk of physical disability
- Decreased strength and need for assistance with normal tasks
- Increased risk of falls
- Increased risk of early death
- Increased insulin resistance and higher risk of Type 2 diabetes
- Decreased energy and quality of life

So, is this really an **age**-related issue? If that's true, we're all sunk as we get older, correct? But let's look at what the data report about age-related muscle loss before we see gloom and doom in our future. Remember how important mindset is? Knowing the facts discourages a fixed mindset of a negative future.

I looked at as many published studies as I could for several weeks and found some very interesting facts. There's a lot of variability in how the studies on sarcopenia were done. Essentially, there was a marked difference in which muscles were assessed, how they were assessed, the people that were studied, and so on.

This variability makes it next to impossible to discover a valid and accurate "cause" of sarcopenia. The lack of consistency makes it difficult to draw conclusions that help us understand what happens, and why, during the aging process in the human body.

There's also a concern many studies have relatively small sample sizes and are using indirect methods for estimating muscle tissue, such as total body potassium. Say what?

Let me share some of the highlights reported in a few of these studies.

Age-related lean muscle loss studies

I've observed the real reason it happens. It's not age. I repeat, it's **not** age. Looking at the details of the studies, age has next to nothing to do with it.

A 12-year study looked at the muscle fiber of the knee and elbow in 12 reportedly healthy, sedentary men. They measured upper and lower body muscle groups initially and then measured nine of them again 12 years later. Decreased strength was seen during the second measurement, particularly in the quadriceps.

Did you notice the most important fact? The specific population studied was **sedentary**. These men *hadn't exercised* in the 12 years since the onset of the study. Who wouldn't lose lean muscle mass when not exercising for 12 years?!

This study stated:[1] *"Our observations suggest that a quantitative loss in muscle cross sectional area is a major contributor to the decrease in muscle strength seen with advancing age and, together with muscle strength at first measurement, accounts for 90% of the variability in strength at second measurement."*

I'm completely dumbfounded that *age* is reported to be the culprit here instead of the elephant in the room. They were S-E-D-E-N-T-A-R-Y!

Even young people weaken without exercise! Stating muscle loss is age-related versus muscle loss is due to not exercising is like comparing air with water. They both contain oxygen, don't they? Are they the same or different? You can't breathe water and you can't drink air.

Another study looked at 12 younger (21–31 years of age) and 12 older (66–78 years of age) subjects. Both groups consisted of six men and six women.

The muscles were measured by assessing how much power and speed could be produced during a contraction of the muscles that bend the ankle and straighten the knee. I looked to see if the older people were sedentary or active. All that was reported regarding their activity levels was a general statement that "all subjects were healthy and ranged from sedentary to recreationally active."

I could find no description of what *recreationally active* meant anywhere in the entire paper.

The findings? There was no difference noted between younger and older groups when assessing ankle strength. There was a difference noted when assessing the thigh muscles that work to straighten the knee. Was this due to being sedentary? It wasn't delineated.

I'll now unveil the term I use instead of *age*-related lean muscle loss. Ready? *Time*-related lean muscle loss. It's a direct response of the body to lack of physical exercise over T-I-M-E. It's not because of age. Now, that's good news!!!

Just so you know, this isn't my opinion. The data bear this fact out. Exercise can be seen as the true fountain of youth!

Men who were studied during their 20s to see how three weeks of bed rest impacted them were studied again in their 50s.[2] They'd lost exercise capacity and gained weight over 30 years BUT exercise was seen to restore what had been lost in just six months! I want to mention, the loss over 30 years was not as much as the three weeks of bed rest caused when they were 20. Bed rest is devastating to muscles. Being a "couch potato" is detrimental to aging well.

The good news is more and more studies are reporting that resistance exercises reverse aging in human skeletal muscles by as much as 50 percent![3,4]

An 86-year-old patient I had many years ago needed assistance to rise from a chair. He'd weakened when he stopped walking to the corner store to get the morning paper. After just a few weeks of strength training, he could leg press 200 pounds and get up out of a chair like a shot! He didn't get younger. He got stronger …

I've seen exercise literally eliminate disability in older adults. I repeat, it's NOT A-G-E!

Before I tell you what Sue thought of me during our first encounter, I'll tell you what I didn't tell her. All my years of experience working with older populations caused me to firmly believe she'd end up not just needing a walker, but likely end up in a nursing home as her needs progressed beyond what her family could do for her.

So, what did Sue say she felt when we first met? She literally hated me. She hated what I had to say about her needing a walker in five years. She hated the whole encounter. But guess what? Sue and I eventually became a mutual admiration society. She agreed to working with me at her husband's urging, and as she felt less and less pain over the weeks that followed and was able to do more and more, she began to see the wisdom of exercise and performing effective self-care methods.

I admired the fact she followed through despite detesting exercise. She did all that was asked of her and reaped the benefits. Sue learned other people could not make her body strong and functional. She needed to do the work.

She also learned there is no magic pill.

PART 2

Common Aging Culprits and Their Victims

I've spent my entire professional life teaching things that are not well known but should be. I'll never forget a woman in one of my Nourish Your Body for Life classes. She looked like a deer in headlights and asked, *"why didn't anyone tell me this before?"*

People Can't Teach What They Don't Know

The reality is people can't share or teach what they don't know. There are many very well meaning, yet misinformed, health care professionals.

An orthopedic surgeon isn't taught impaired ankle function inhibits proper knee performance. He will see something on an X-ray or MRI and recommend surgery to address what's found. That's what he's trained to do.

A cardiologist was not taught what damages endothelial cell function. She'll prescribe medications to manipulate high blood pressure and high cholesterol, not understanding this won't repair injured cells or prevent heart attacks or strokes by more than 3 percent.

A pelvic floor specialist isn't taught about the connection between the pelvic floor and hip rotator muscles and the benefits of training in weight-bearing exercise. Treatments and exercises may or may not work well to enable the pelvic floor muscles to support a full bladder without unwanted leakage.

You Must Be Informed

I'm not saying to not take prescribed medications. I'm not saying to never have surgery. I am saying you must be fully informed of the risks and benefits of any treatments. You must be informed of what's known to cause the things that get medically or surgically manipulated. You must be informed of what is known to work, even if it's not mainstream knowledge. Being informed leads to better decisions and improved outcomes.

Being informed is necessary to radically increase your odds of living well as long as you are above ground.

CHAPTER 5

Disposable Underwear, Anyone?

MYTH: Unwanted urine leakage is a rite of passage as you age.

Joyce went to *a specialist who prescribed medication to treat her urinary incontinence. Her symptoms persisted, and eventually she sought a second opinion. Joyce was recommended for surgery at that point. You'll never guess what she was told by the surgeon!*

I'll finish Joyce's story after providing much-needed education that's not mainstream knowledge but should be. Even most pelvic floor experts are unaware of what you'll learn in this chapter.

For those over the age of 65 and still living at home, more than 50 percent of women and 25 percent of men report urinary incontinence,[1] but this matter is much more serious than just buying disposable underwear. Urinary incontinence has a profound impact on the quality of life of older people,[2] their subjective health status,[3] and levels of depression.[4] Incontinence intimately impacts the need for care[5] as family members are challenged to provide proper hygiene, ultimately requiring placement of loved ones in facilities, causing guilt and heartbreak to all involved.

Is incontinence really a "normal" rite of passage as you age? Can you not go below ground without having experienced the embarrassment of leaking when you cough?

Have you seen those commercials that show a woman getting dressed for a date as she shows off a "pretty" pair of disposable underwear? The intention of the ad is to show that a woman can be both beautiful and sexy while essentially wearing an adult diaper. Really?! Like anyone EVER *felt* beautiful OR sexy when they sneezed and leaked urine! REALLY?!

"Needing disposable underwear as I age is my personal goal," said no one ever! Just sayin'.

Because we all want a happy and healthy life without the need for disposable underwear as we age, it's critical to gain an understanding of true pelvic floor function to address this problem effectively.

UI is nothing new. Historical records show male UI was mentioned as far back as 500 B.C. in Egyptian manuscripts.[6] Current devices for male incontinence are modeled after those first created in 1747. You'd think we'd be a little more advanced by now ... but this is not a 21st century problem. It's been around a long time.

Kegel Exercises

Despite this problem not being anything new, the subject was never exactly a conversation starter at social gatherings. Arnold Kegel, MD, deserves the most credit for bringing this topic out into the open as many felt too ashamed to even tell their doctor. Dr. Kegel, an American gynecologist, developed a device that measured the contraction strength of the muscles supporting pelvic organs. The device was designed to assist with specific exercises seen to improve prolapse and UI issues.

While we're very grateful for Dr. Kegel's contribution, there's a lot more to the story than Kegel exercises when it comes to stopping unwanted leakage. Yes, there are times Kegel exercises help to improve symptoms. This is why they're so highly recommended, and there are countless online resources teaching them. However, as many reading this may attest to, Kegel exercises don't always work. If they did, we wouldn't have entire aisles of adult diaper options in all the grocery, drug, and big-box stores.

The main premise of performing Kegel exercises is to consciously squeeze your "bathroom" muscles with the intention of strengthening the muscles so unwanted urine leakage doesn't happen.

Kegel exercises focus on strengthening the external urethral sphincter muscles so you can keep it closed until it's safe to urinate. The urethra is the tube whereby urine exits the body from the bladder. Your internal sphincter is involuntary, which means you have no control over its function. Your external sphincter is voluntary, which means it allows conscious control over when urine exits your body.

The goal with Kegel exercises is to improve this conscious control by strengthening the ability to contract and keep the sphincter closed until you're safely on the toilet.

BUT … *Your Pelvic Floor Is Much More Than a Sphincter* …

First off, floor isn't really accurate because it's more of a bowl, but floor is the term everyone knows so I will use that for simplicity. A healthy pelvic floor is designed to successfully support the organs positioned above it, including bladder, prostate for men, uterus for women, and bowel. A healthy, well functioning pelvic floor supports a full, heavy bladder without leaking even when there's no bathroom in sight.

The major player providing this support is the levator ani muscle, further defined as puborectalis, pubococcygeus, and iliococcygeus.

Urinary incontinence is not the only result of poor muscle support. Organ prolapses can also result because the levator ani is designed to provide a force forward toward the pubic bone and upward to keep organs properly positioned. This means the bladder, uterus, and rectum can all drop down from weak support.

The main reason Kegel exercises often fail is because you can't consciously squeeze your levator ani muscle and improve its ability to support all those organs, including a full, heavy bladder. Imagine if you could restore functional strength in your body just by squeezing muscles when you think about them. No one would ever have to go to the gym again!

The levator ani muscle is designed to work *subconsciously*, without thinking about it. You can squeeze your bathroom muscles till the cows come home, but if your levator ani is not strong enough to support the weight of up to 2 cups of urine, you'll be buying disposable underwear before you know it.

If you've searched mainstream information or consulted with a health care professional, either or both sources may lack understanding of just how much everything is connected to everything else. Because the world has a seriously bad habit of isolating systems and body parts, this is a stumbling block to success because you don't take your pelvis off (or any other body part) and put it on a shelf when you go to bed.

EVERYTHING IS CONNECTED TO EVERYTHING ELSE.

Let's define some things and look more closely at whole body anatomy to better understand the potential causes of this often socially debilitating experience. My goal is to help you become more informed.

Types of Incontinence

There are four basic types of urinary incontinence: urge, stress, overflow or retention, and mixed.

Urge incontinence is when you have almost no time to get to the toilet before unwanted leakage occurs. Falls are not uncommon when this happens as a bathroom floor can be slippery when wet!

Stress incontinence is when leakage happens while sneezing, coughing, or physically exerting yourself. It often happens when jumping on a trampoline. Many a person has been caught off guard when this happens for the first time, and you can always tell by the look on their face! I remember a study concluding that trampoline training increased risk of incontinence because so many young women experienced this problem. They have it backward. The trampoline exposes the existing weak pelvic floor. Yes, young people can have this issue too.

Overflow incontinence (urinary retention) leads to dripping and occurs when you're unable to fully empty your bladder. There is chronic and acute retention. Acute retention can be life-threatening, requiring immediate medical attention. This is the most common urologic emergency in males, yet is a rare occurrence in females. I've had homecare patients who used intermittent catheterization to empty their bladders several times a day because of urinary retention.

Mixed incontinence includes both stress and urge. You'll feel the need to rush to the bathroom to avoid an accident AND you'll notice unwanted leakage when physically active, sneezing, or coughing.

Reported Causes of UI

Mainstream reported causes of UI include a very long list of things including urinary tract infections, constipation, alcohol or caffeine intake, heart/blood pressure meds, sedatives, muscle relaxers, high doses of Vitamin C intake, obesity, nerve damage, enlarged prostate, overactive bladder muscles, menopause, and pregnancy.

Whew! That's a LOT of *potential* causes. Another reason to check the side effects of your medications. Don't you think it's funny how so many people can drink all the coffee they want and not be incontinent? Isn't it weird how not EVERY post-menopausal woman is incontinent? Why is that?! Why on Earth would a bladder become overactive?! Why does a prostate become enlarged? What CAUSES these things?

When I see a patient with a diagnosis of tendonitis, I always ask, "why is the tendon inflamed?" To me it's better to address the CAUSE and not just treat the symptom. I believe the same thing is important when looking at UI.

From what I've seen over the years of working with people, there is a common cause that's not well known, even by clinical experts.

Although someone can have nerve damage or other serious issues, most often it's something related to physical function. Let me tell you what they didn't tell you, because they didn't know. It may due to *everything being connected to everything else.*

The Pelvic Floor Is Connected to ...

As stated earlier, it's not really a floor. The shape is more like a deep bowl.

You were introduced to the muscles that make up the pelvic floor already. The levator ani muscles are the major player, but what you'll probably NOT hear from any clinician or medical expert is the fact that the levator ani muscles have a fascial connection to the obturator internus muscle. The obturator internus is a hip rotation muscle that directly impacts the function of the pelvic floor because of the fascial connection.

Why does that fascial connection matter?

Because the fascial connection from the hip rotator stimulates the pelvic muscles to do their job when you're upright, weight-bearing, and using your hip muscles.

In your real-life context, your hip function directly impacts your pelvic floor function.

Guess what happens if your hips weaken due to injury or being non-weight-bearing from a knee or ankle issue or from years of prolonged sitting? Your obturator internus stops stimulating your levator ani muscle and strength in the pelvic floor decreases slowly and steadily. Then one day, without warning, you cough or sneeze or jump and wham! You leak. Or one day you feel the urge to go to the bathroom and shocker, you leak BEFORE you get to the toilet!

If you've ever been to a pelvic floor specialist, I'll bet you were never told about the connection of your pelvic floor to your hip muscles. People can't teach what they don't know.

Whenever I worked with someone post hip replacement, I'd impress upon them the importance of restoring full hip function to reduce their risk of needing disposable underwear in their future. They were my most compliant patients ever!

If you've ever been non-weight-bearing because of an injury or surgery, your pelvic floor function has probably been affected. Maybe you're not noticing any symptoms … yet …

Scientific studies back this up. Being sedentary[7,8] is directly related to increased prevalence of incontinence. Sitting on your backside for hours every day weakens your hips and, ultimately, your pelvic floor function. Anyone completely wheelchair-bound or bed-bound will have issues with incontinence.

A healthy bladder can hold just over 1 pound of liquid, which puts pressure on the supporting muscles. Weak muscles can't hold the bladder up in its proper position. As the bladder drops down, it pulls open the sphincter you're desperately trying to hold closed until it's safe to go to the bathroom.

How Everything Is Connected to Everything Else

Teaching how everything is connected to everything else is one of my favorite things to do. It's also where so many lack knowledge and understanding. You're not a bladder that walks in the door OR a sphincter. You're a whole person, and you'll now learn how even your ankles can impact the function of your pelvic floor. Did I just write ankles?! Yes, ankles …

Your ankles and your pelvic floor

If you have decreased motion in your ankle, it will affect pretty much every joint in your body when moving in weight-bearing positions, including pelvic floor function. A whole-body reaction occurs from the foot up that either supports pain-free function or leads to dysfunction over time. I always assess ankle function in everyone who's able to walk. I also teach this fact in all my movement classes.

Do you have a history of ankle sprains?

Your trunk and your pelvic floor

Limitations in your thoracic spine, between your neck and low back, can lead to your respiratory diaphragm not loading symmetrically. Why does this matter? Your diaphragm isometrically impacts the loading and exploding of your pelvic floor. If there's impaired motion in your rib cage, your diaphragm will be affected and, ultimately, your pelvic floor. Your hips also rely on trunk rotation to provide stimulation for optimal hip rotation. Many people have limited trunk motion.

Do you struggle to turn and see when backing up your car?

Your hips and your pelvic floor

Limitations in one or both hips can affect pelvic floor muscles, causing them to be "switched off." Your pelvic floor muscles are stimulated by hip rotation. Total hip replacements can cause decreased hip rotation. Either the painful hip prior to surgery inhibits function or the post-surgical restoration to full function is lacking. This can lead to incontinence, which can improve or worsen after surgery depending on your situation.

The good news is that all these areas can be improved with the right whole-body conditioning done the right way!

What to Do About It

Given that your pelvic floor muscles are required to support your bladder as it fills with urine and gets heavier, isn't it important to train those muscles in the way they actually function?

What do I mean by that? Because the levator ani muscles function subconsciously, you can't *consciously* squeeze your bathroom muscles to restore optimal function. You must MOVE your body in a way that causes the muscles to subconsciously REACT to the movement.

This means training while on your feet, working your hips and trunk. If you have a history of an ankle sprain or have been non-weight-bearing for any reason; you may also want to specifically assess and target your ankle function in weight-bearing.

Because teaching movement correctly, with recommended modifications to meet potential deficits, lacks accuracy in written form, I provide a video link in Resources.

The best way to stimulate and strengthen the levator ani muscles is to work the hip rotation muscles in weight-bearing. Because the pelvic floor is an important part of the pelvic core, sports performance is also enhanced with this type of focused training. I've had students in my classes report their running performance improved from this type of training and conditioning. Many also reported improved knee or low back pain!

It's important to emphasize modifications are necessary if there are balance issues or any existing limited function due to joint pain. Please seek an expert to be sure you don't hurt yourself or aggravate an existing condition. But when doing the right training for these muscles, improvements are often seen in just a few weeks. Having taught many classes for this problem, I've seen some report improvement in as little as one week! Of course, results vary based on the person's specific circumstances.

Ready to learn what Joyce was told during her consultation with the second expert? She was told the medication she'd been prescribed was useless for the type of UI she had and if she'd been taught exercises at that time, she may have been able to avoid surgery.

He informed her that surgery was her only viable option at this point as her bladder had dropped to the point of no return without surgical intervention. She now needed a colposuspension surgery to resolve her UI. Ouch!!!

If you spend copious amounts of time sitting, you must train to develop healthy pelvic floor function. It won't happen by default.

There's no magic pill. Aging well requires active work. Aging well doesn't happen by default.

Hopefully, you now understand incontinence is not an age-related issue; it's a mobility- and strength-related issue. There's no magic pill that restores healthy pelvic floor function. Medical interventions may address some of the symptoms, but they don't restore proper strength to the pelvic floor OR the human body. Thankfully, the right training can.

CHAPTER 6

Weebles Wobble and They Might Fall Down . . .

MYTH: Instability comes with age.

Assistive Devices

The use of canes, walkers, and wheelchairs is prevalent in the older population. Are these required to decrease the risk of falls because of age? Is it age or some other reason?

Let me begin by asking a very important question. Did you know a cane, walker, or a wheelchair will not *prevent* falls and injuries?! Are you surprised? I've been up close and personal to those who use these devices. I've seen people become injured from a fall while using them. Yes, even wheelchairs!

How can this happen? Aren't these devices designed to prevent falls? NO! That's a misconception. Concern over a beloved family member with poor balance leads many to believe they'll be safe once they obtain a cane or a walker. This isn't true. They may be safer, or they may not.

When someone has poor stability, they'll simply fall WITH their assistive device. The cane or walker will NOT keep them upright. Even a wheelchair won't prevent all falls. I've seen people lean forward from their wheelchair to pick something up off the floor and fall out of the chair. Of course, I didn't stand by and watch them fall! When someone is found on the floor in front of their wheelchair by staff or family members, they'll typically say they were trying to pick something up that they dropped.

So, what's a cane, walker, or wheelchair supposed to do? They're assistive devices which means their role is to *assist* with getting someone from point A to point B. They assist mobility. That's all. Yes, many well meaning health care professionals advise someone to get a cane or walker, perhaps thinking that will make them safer. Assistive devices may provide a margin of safety that isn't there without the device, but this is only if it's due to weakness or fatigue with walking. The device is meant to help support body weight or decrease pain from weight-bearing. No assistive device holds people up if they lose their balance.

A cane decreases weight-bearing on one side of the body and provides a "third leg," if you will, for a little more stability. If your left leg is weak or has a painful knee, a cane in your right hand will offset or decrease the amount of support the left leg needs to provide. Many use a cane on the wrong side thinking that's the side they want to help. This places more weight and requires more work on the side the cane is used. To be clear, a cane will not *prevent* falls that occur due to impaired stability or severe weakness.

A walker, with or without wheels, provides support if a person has weakness or tires easily when walking from their recliner to the kitchen sink for example. Which type of walker you use makes a difference. Many think the wheels might make a person less stable, yet picking up a standard walker to move it forward to take the next step can cause someone with balance deficits to lose their balance and fall. In this case, the wheeled walker is a safer choice.

Because 40 percent of older adults living at home experience a fall once a year[1] and fall rates in facilities are even higher,[2] it seems we need to be looking at what we can do about it.

Yes, falls in nursing homes happen quite often. I know because I worked in one for nearly a decade. Due to laws that strictly prohibit restraints of any kind, residents with dementia are free to stand up from their wheelchairs and walk, even if they aren't safe to do so. Staff then do their best to encourage them to sit back down. It's a common nursing home dilemma.

Restraints cover a surprising multitude of things, including footrests as they can impede the person from standing. I know, I know. It makes little sense, and the staff in these facilities are constantly running to support a resident who gets up and is at risk of falling. Even tray tables are considered a restraint if the resident can't independently move it out of the way to stand.

These facts may seem confusing because they put a person at increased risk of falling, but please understand, I've been in my profession long enough to remember posey vests. They were likened to a strait jacket that literally tied a patient to their wheelchair to prevent standing up and falling. Of course, if this is your beloved parent tied to a chair, you may be glad restraints have been abolished. Yet, to prevent any potential misuse or abuse of restraints, things have gone too far the other way, with more falls now happening to those at risk.

Even bedrails are considered a restraint! You may be shocked to learn that residents at risk of falling are now in beds lowered as close to the floor as possible with cushioned mats placed on the floor on both sides of the bed in case they roll out. Bedrails are considered potentially dangerous as they can trap an arm or a head. Special paperwork must be filled out to allow a facility to provide bedrails to a resident needing assistance to sit up independently.

Sadly, the use of mobility devices has been increasing over the past few decades.[3] A 2020 study published in *BMC Geriatrics* reported the use of walking aids issued to older adults to prevent falls has been identified as a risk factor.[4] Yes, using a walker can literally *increase* the risk of falls. Part of the reason for this is incorrect use due to environmental constraints. This means their bathroom may be too small to navigate a walker safely, so unsafe strategies like lifting the walker while walking sideways are used when needing to use the toilet.

When working in homecare, I saw many issues in home environments that made proper, safe use of a mobility device impossible. We worked out other strategies like installing grab bars and so on, but many people don't have an expert in their home to advise them.

It's imperative to have a professional assess a person's gait and ability to get around with the correct mobility device for them and educate them in its proper use. Unfortunately, many people purchase a device for themselves or a loved one and have no idea how to use it safely or if it's even the correct device for their needs. I've seen health care professionals tell a patient to get a cane without the thought they may not know how to use it correctly.

Balance and Stability

Let's now look at the difference between balance and stability. Yes, they're different. Balance is the ability to maintain a position. I expect you have tried standing on one leg and counting to 10 or 30 …

That's balance. It's maintaining the position. Stability is much more than that. Stability is the ability to regain a position once it's been disrupted. People fall if they can't regain their position once it's been disrupted, even if they can stand on one leg for 30 seconds.

Example: A person is walking down the hallway, and someone calls their name. They turn to see who it is, and they fall. Their upright position while walking was disrupted by turning and they couldn't regain that position. This happens even with a walker. So, training to improve stability is key. Standing on one leg for 30 seconds will not improve *stability.*

Stability strategically enhances all that we do.

Stability must be trained in motion, not stillness. Stability is not rigidity. Stability is fluidity with control. Notice if standing on one leg causes you to become stiff and rigid to keep your balance. People don't typically fall when they are standing still. It happens when they're moving. So, doesn't it make sense to train for stability with movement?

Let's clarify.

Stability: The property of a body that causes it, when disturbed from a condition of equilibrium or steady motion, to develop forces or moments that restore the original condition. Sounds like being able to *restore* balance when lost or challenged, doesn't it?

Balance: The ability to move or to remain in a position without losing control or falling. One could argue being stable with good balance is to fully function in the daily tasks of life and NOT FALL DOWN.

Okay, let's move past semantics and into what really matters. How does our body maintain or regain stability while performing functional tasks like walking and dancing? Why do some lose it and fall? More importantly can we restore it once it becomes impaired?

This is a matter of great importance because the statistics are quite sobering. Falls are reported by the CDC to be the greatest health risk among people 65 and older. Ouch! Sadly, falls are also the *leading cause* of fatal injuries for older Americans. Since I teach on how to age well without decline, it would seem NOT losing stability as you age is a necessary goal to achieve that end.

Hospital for Special Surgery's VOICES 60+ Senior Advocacy Program provides details about where these falls occur:[5]

- 60 percent of falls happen inside the home
- 30 percent of falls occur outside the home, like while shopping or walking
- 10 percent occur in a health care center such as a hospital, clinic, or nursing/rehabilitation facility

More sobering statistics from the CDC include:[6]

- One in four adults falls each day
- 20 to 30 percent who fall sustain a serious injury
- 850,000 who fall are hospitalized each year
- 29,000 die each year from falls

To be fair, many elderly people die after a fall (if not immediately from the fall) because of poor health and multiple health issues they had BEFORE they fell. The fall was simply the last straw OR their body was failing, and they were ready to pass away, fall or no fall.

I have seen many active elderly people recover well from a fall and resume their lives. That said, no one wants to fall, and the fear of falling exponentially impacts quality of life and often inhibits being active.

Let's look at why certain strategies work and others don't when it comes to improving stability.

There are three components to balance. Yes, I'm using the term balance here because a person can have trouble maintaining a position in stillness if they have issues with any of these three components. Have you ever been so dizzy you couldn't stand up? Have you noticed when you close your eyes, you begin to sway a little just standing still?

The three main components to balance are:

- Vestibular (inner ear)
- Visual
- Proprioceptive (whole body communication)

I'll briefly mention the first two, and then focus on the proprioceptive component. My goal is not to create a scientific tome here, but simply relate facts you may find helpful. Other systems, such as cerebellar, vestibulocochlear, and vascular/vasovagal systems, are also known players in balance but let's keep this simple.

It's important you're aware that dizziness or vertigo is a common side effect of many medications in case this is the cause for you or a loved one. Did you read chapter 2? Knowing this is critical so you can discuss options with your prescribing practitioner.

Vestibular

Vestibular function resides in your inner ear, with data showing impaired hearing is a risk factor for falling.[7,8]

I'm sure many of you remember when you rode an amusement park ride that spun you around, and how you felt dizzy when you stopped. I used to get the teacup spinning so fast my daughters and I were a blur to my husband as he watched. He was fond of saying just watching us made him nauseous. The simple explanation of why dizziness happens is because the fluid in the inner ear continues to move crystals positioned there after you stop moving.

There's also an inner ear dysfunction that can lead to benign paroxysmal positional vertigo (BPPV), which is a case of those crystals shifting into the wrong place. This is successfully treated using the Epley Maneuver or another method. Please seek out expert guidance to ensure you're doing the right thing(s) for your symptoms.

Visual

Your eyes provide a visual reference of your physical position in space, and so typically, the reason impaired vision increases the risk of falls is due to not seeing, or tripping on, environmental hazards. Things such as area rugs not lying flat, missing a step height, and so on. Most of these falls tend to happen at night when the light is dim as well, decreasing visual acuity.

That said, research shows eliminating visual cues to body position by closing the eyes is seen to increase body sway by a factor of three. This means vision loss can impact how your body knows where it is in space. Your balance mechanisms literally create movement to figure out where we are in space. Fascinating, don't you think?

Conversely, those who have vestibular AND proprioceptive deficits rely more heavily on vision, and if the balance system doesn't adapt to increased reliance on vision, balance may be more compromised. Postural stability is known to be adversely affected by impaired vision.[9]

Vestibular and visual systems work in tandem from birth. It's the vestibular system that guides your balance, which in turn guides the development of your vision during your first years after birth. This means when we're young, movement guides vision. However, as soon as we develop the necessary visual skills, vision begins to guide balance. Wow, are we complex beings or what?

Your vision is such a powerful sense it can override information from the other senses, which is sometimes beneficial and other times detrimental. If the visual system is not working properly, it can provide incorrect information to other somatosensory systems.

Sadly, many people develop impaired vision as they age (cataracts, macular degeneration, and so on), which in turn can impair balance. Fortunately, neuroplasticity allows your brain to continuously create new pathways and neurological connections, which allows you to develop improved control over different sensory systems.

Neuroplasticity is why blind people who were not born that way don't lose their balance when walking or dancing or moving. This is also why proper training and education for the elderly can improve balance, despite visual deficits no matter your age. More on that next.

Proprioceptive

Proprioception is the information perceived through your muscles, joints, and fascia to tell your brain where you are in space.

Proprioceptors organize coordinated movement by "turning muscles on" when movement occurs. The muscles' job is then to control the movement. If you've heard me speak, you probably remember my mention of eccentric control. Eccentric control is when a muscle lengthens under tension to control motion. Proprioceptors play a colossal role in that ability.

Healthy proprioceptive ability is tantamount to not only knowing where you are in space, but also knowing when your balance is challenged and how to regain it if lost. This is HUGE regarding healthy stability and decreasing the risk of falls.

Three groups of proprioceptors reside in

- joint capsules and ligaments
- muscles, tendons, and tendinous junctions
- fascial complexes and skin

In these groups, there are nine different types of proprioceptors, each responding differently to velocity (speed) changes, such as whether there is acceleration or deceleration. They also respond uniquely based on how much mechanical force is occurring, with a different threshold required for each.

The phenomenal complexities and intricacies of the human body continue to challenge our understanding, but we've come a long way in recent years as we've teased out these differences, including how they affect our physical movement and function.

If you'd like to know all the glorious details about specific proprioceptors, Resources shows where you can find more content.

What's key to know? Proprioceptors are subconscious reactors, not conscious actors. They rely on authentic movement to be "fed," not starved out or inhibited by isolated movement training. This means isolating muscles when exercising does not improve proprioceptive function.

Fine-tuning your training to ensure ALL your proprioceptors are engaged authentically in motion is key.

Things like surgery, immobilization, pain, weakness, poor range of motion, compensation, poor training, poor tissue integrity, and so on can all inhibit proprioceptive function.

Are you ready to learn what have been shown to be the BEST ways to restore balance when impaired as well as how to enhance the function of proprioceptors? Hint: it's not done when lying down OR training on a wobble board. Surprise!

The more you understand why you're doing something, the more apt you are to actually DO IT. This breeds success!

Please remember that stability strategically enhances all we do. Your center of gravity (COG) shifts to trigger stability, which is why it's critical to be trained in motion, not stillness. Standing on one leg for a prolonged period will not stimulate your proprioceptors. Remember, healthy balance that reduces fall risk isn't rigidity, it's fluidity with control.

How far forward can you reach without losing control? Can you turn around without grabbing for support?

Motion is what turns on proprioceptors. Proprioceptors then turn on muscles. Based on 30 years of experience, the most effective way to ensure enhanced function doesn't decline is to train in all three planes of motion while on your feet. Couple this training with successful, competent repetitions and you develop *efficient, stable motion.*

If compensatory mechanisms (your body "cheating" to get the task done) are present, it's important to tweak movements outside proprioceptors' preferred patterns while also ensuring you're building safely on success. If movement lacks confidence and requires extraneous motions to provide safety, it's unlikely to improve the authentic proprioceptive function that is the goal. If you compensate while training, you're strengthening your dysfunction! Your brain will cheat to keep you safe, and you won't even know it.

Training where the body changes direction can be key but MUST be within your threshold of success. The goal is to prevent overloading the structures you desire to improve. You can BUILD on your success when training without compensation, but you cannot create success out of a dysfunctional movement pattern.

Three-Plane Function for Stability

Ensuring your body moves and stabilizes in all three planes of motion is the most effective way to reduce your risk of physically aging with decline. It's also the most effective way I have seen in all my years of working with older populations. It works for those from 9 years old to 99 years old and older!

When your ankles work as designed, your proprioceptors are prompted at the right time in the right way, so your muscles respond the way they were designed to respond. When your hips work as designed, your pelvis and center of gravity are in the right place at the right time with active movement. I cannot emphasize enough how important this is, not just for balance, but for common pain patterns as well.

I teach stability classes on a regular basis, and I have videos on my YouTube channel that provide some training for this topic. Check Resources for details.

Then, there came the autopilot.

In the MELT Method® world, per Sue Hitzmann's impressive knowledge of the neurofascial system, "autopilot" is a term used for a jaw-dropping array of communication that occurs with both dynamic and static balance. In one of her blogs, she describes three nets of connection comprised of circulatory, fascial, and neural systems.[10] You may be fascinated to learn (I was, geek that I am) the differences in speed in which these systems function.

Your circulatory system is quite slow, relatively speaking. It takes a full 90 seconds for a red blood cell to travel out from and return back to your heart.

Your nervous system functions with varied speeds from 7 to 170 miles per hour, which appears fast with a capital F, but the fascial system wins hands down. It literally functions near the speed of sound at 720 miles per hour!

I've seen MELT Method techniques improve balance in some of the most challenging issues, including Parkinson's and post-stroke patients. This is why I have been teaching it, and benefiting personally by it, since 2011.

Clinical studies on balance

A 2019 review[11] that consisted of 22 studies and 200 subjects, average age 75 years, reported the effects observed on static and dynamic balance using many different approaches, including:

- resistance and aerobic exercise
- balance training
- T-bow©
- wobble board training
- aerobic step
- stability ball training
- adapted physical activity
- Wii Fit training

Training times varied from 10 minutes twice a week up to 90 minutes three times a week.

Balance tests/retests consisted of the following:

- timed up and go
- Berg balance
- one-leg stance
- Tinetti

- unipedal
- Wii Fit tests

All these tests varied with the intervention being assessed.

What I found most interesting was the fact ALL intervention groups, regardless of the activity performed, saw improvement in balance, and ALL control groups (no exercise) saw a decline in balance, no matter which tests were used to assess it.

The common factor in the intervention groups was an increase in strength. Those that engaged in both aerobic type activity and exercise saw more improvement than either type of activity performed alone. So, is it inactivity or loss of joint function or speed of movement or … that leads to balance deficits over time? It seems the most important factor is NOT being sedentary.

None of these study results confirmed or refuted any specific activity or exercise when it comes to improving balance.

So, what does this mean? This means studies haven't found the "Holy Grail" for balance exercises yet. This doesn't mean there aren't any that succeed more than others. Sadly, they didn't compare three-plane eccentric loading or the MELT Method in their studies. In my humble opinion based on experience, they would have seen superior results had they included these two methods in the clinical trials. This is what I've seen in my practice for many years, no matter the age or issues of the person training.

There are so many structures involved in balance that we may never understand it fully. The most important fact about balance and risk of falls is this: increasing strength and activity levels show a linear improvement in balance. Conversely, inactivity and weakness lead to an increase in falls.

Movement matters … there is no magic pill.

CHAPTER 7

Stairs or No Stairs, That Is the Question

MYTH: Joint pain is normal.

I'll never forget coming across an ad while researching for the Reverse Aging Boot Camp. The ad was aimed at real estate professionals and focused on the need for people literally "aging out" of their homes. Not because they need care, but because they need a living environment without stairs or other areas that require being physically capable of living in them. Wow! Doesn't that just say it all?!

Reams of online articles speak of how to "age in place" by having a home without stairs: *"For seniors seeking age-friendly housing options or families looking to future-proof their abode against potential mobility issues down the line, zero-entry homes (no stairs, wide doorways, etc.) present an ideal solution."*[1]

Another sad statement: *"Make sure your home is built for aging in place. A large home with lots of stairs may not be a good fit as you get older. Make it a place that you will live in for the rest of your life …"*[2]

And another: *"Many homeowners today plan to age in place, and having a home without stairs makes that easier."*[3]

I'm about to tell you this isn't a "normal" future. It may be *common*, but it is NOT a *normal* aspect of aging. Let's delve into some of the reasons this occurs and, of course, cover the most important part: what you can do about it!

The main reasons people have trouble navigating stairs include weakness, poor balance, and joint pain. There may be some medical conditions or post-surgical issues, but for the most part, those are the top three reasons. Since I cover balance and strength elsewhere, I'll focus on *joint pain* in this chapter.

Joint Pain

Much of what causes joint pain has next to nothing to do with OA. Yes, many people have joint damage that is confirmed via imaging with an X-ray or MRI. I'm not saying people don't have OA.

Let me explain by sharing a story.

Marge came into the clinic with a complaint of right knee pain. Her prescription gave a diagnosis of right knee OA. After getting a detailed history and assessing her three-plane whole body function in weight-bearing movement, it was obvious her left ankle lacked function in both range of motion and stability. Marge shared that she'd sprained that ankle years ago, but it had seemed to recover okay. She hadn't ever had any treatment for it.

Marge was completely unaware there were deficits in her ankle function. This is because our brains are notorious for not telling us when we have an issue with motion or stability somewhere if it doesn't cause pain. The problem arises when the compensations caused by the deficit begin to annoy and injure structures not designed to do what they're being asked to do because of the deficit.

Marge's knee was being stressed because it was having to do what it wasn't designed for in order to make up for the deficit in the ankle. She questioned how her left ankle could cause pain in her right knee. A fair question. Let's look at how we walk to answer this question.

The complexities of gait are far too numerous to cover in depth here, but I'll attempt to share a basic understanding that doesn't make your eyes glaze over if you're not a lover of science and biomechanics like me.

When you take a step and land on your heel, your foot reacts with a specific joint motion that causes a flexible, shock-absorbing action as your foot begins to take on your body weight.

That specific ankle joint motion, along with physics, creates a reaction from your ankle to your shin, thigh, hip, pelvis, and all the way to your trunk.

That reaction then creates a response, the opposite reaction, from your trunk all the way back down to your ankle, causing you to push off your toe with a solid, stable foot action to take the next step.

This happens from the time you land on your heel to the time you push off your toes ... with EVERY SINGLE step! Amazing, don't you think?

What happens on one side (foot/leg) intimately impacts what happens on the other side. This is exactly the reason I constantly state *everything is connected to everything else* in my book, *Pain Culprits!* This means it was logical that Marge's left ankle deficits were impacting her right knee function whenever she took a step with either foot.

Because this explanation of joint motion made sense to Marge, we worked to restore left ankle motion and stability with whole body exercises and homework in weight bearing that didn't cause knee pain. Her homework was designed to breed success with no pain and progressed as she improved. The results of her therapy are reported at the end of this chapter, but first I want to address something you may be thinking about right now.

Am I saying if you have severe joint damage, you can magically resolve pain when you walk? No. I'm saying it doesn't cause harm, and just may benefit you, to assess your three-plane function. See if there's another body part aside from where you feel the pain that may be the culprit causing your pain. You can access the Movement Performance Assessment in Resources.

So often the "culprit" causing the pain is not where the "victim" experiencing the pain lives in your body. This means what shows up in your imaging may not be the cause of your pain.

Before you agree to surgery, if it's safe to wait a little bit, shouldn't you see if there's a "culprit" that can be uncovered and corrected?! The downside to not trying this approach is what if the surgery didn't "fix" the pain because it was "caused" by another body part? Ouch!

Stairs and Pain

Stairs are not like walking down the block because you need to raise your body weight when going up or lower your body weight with control when going down. Stairs can be a real nightmare when joint pain occurs.

Going down?

I've worked with many people who experienced knee pain going downstairs, and the problem was limited ankle range of motion. Yes, ankle range of motion must be healthy to not stress your knee as you descend stairs.

Serious joint limitations can sometimes be the cause. Your knee must bend at least 110 degrees to navigate the lowering of your body down a step or a curb without having to turn sideways or perform any physical contortions. It's common to have pain going downstairs after a knee replacement if the range is less than 110 degrees of flexion.

Often, when homecare patients would have enough knee motion and still have pain, I found their ankle function most often to be the culprit. We worked to restore the necessary motion in the ankle and voila! They could now descend stairs without pain or problems.

This means the answer to your knee pain on stairs just may lie in training your ankle the right way. Who knew?

Another issue that can lead to pain when descending stairs is how well your kneecap tracks as your knee bends. Do you remember that commercial from long ago about English muffins with all those nooks and crannies? That's kind of what the back of your kneecap looks like. This is so it can line up perfectly with the structures behind it as your knee bends and straightens.

This problem is so important I posted a YouTube video showing how to check tracking in just a few minutes. You'll find this in Resources.

Decades ago, during a course from Jennifer McConnell, I learned how to apply specialized tape to improve the tracking of the patella. When done the right way for the right reasons, knee pain no longer occurs when going up and down stairs, squatting, or kneeling. That's only if the pain was due to a tracking issue.

Taping also enabled specific exercises, pain-free, to restore muscle function over the course of a couple of weeks. The tape was then no longer needed. McConnell's taping methods also work to treat painful shoulder issues and other areas.

My knowledge back then didn't include understanding just how much everything is connected to everything else. I didn't know at the time just how impactful training the back hip could be at improving patellar tracking, and the best part is there's no taping required.

Although the tape was hypoallergenic and I always applied cover tape under it to further reduce irritation, it still occasionally irritated the skin behind the knee and created a sore spot or two. There were also those who could not be taped at all due to allergies.

If you have trouble descending stairs, how's your ankle function? How's your back hip? I'm talking about Max (gluteus maximus). Have you been sitting on Max for decades, causing progressive weakness? Have you ever assessed Max in three-plane function?

Going up?

Another way back hip dysfunction causes problems is when you're ascending stairs. Pain in your hip, knee, or back when you are going up, not down, can be a sign of back hip dysfunction. Yes, there can always be structural issues that appear on X-ray; however, ensuring the back hip is trained in effective three-plane function, fully mobile, and fully stabile can radically improve your chances of climbing stairs with less pain, maybe even none.

Your back hip is your power source for all things when you're on your feet. I can't tell you how many people have reported increased strength and decreased pain climbing stairs after they began three-plane training.

When you raise your body on a stair, your foot pushes into the stairs with an equal force required to raise your body weight up so the other foot can reach the next stair. The only way the foot can push into the stairs with enough power to raise your bodyweight is if your back hip is capable of that amount of force.

Force must first be loaded to be unloaded. Think of a slingshot. The more you pull the rubber band back, the more force it uses to propel the object forward when you release it. It unloads the force that it first loaded. Your power source works in a similar fashion. It first loads to unload.

YOU NEED STAIRS!

I don't mean to holler at you in all caps, but I really want to get your attention. Yes, you NEED stairs as you get older. You NEED regular exercise to your power source throughout the day, especially if you sit a lot. When you sit a lot, Max gets weak UNLESS you actively train to keep Max strong.

What happens when you decide it's best to live in an environment that requires no physical activity on your part to live there? Everything on one floor and no stairs. One word ... DECLINE.

Decline can suck the joy right out of your life. Without your power source working unimpaired, you'll have trouble sitting down without plopping. You'll have trouble pushing open heavy doors. You'll have trouble getting out of the car without assistance. You'll struggle to pick something up from the floor. You'll need help when stepping off a curb to cross a street. There's more, but I'll stop now before it gets too depressing.

No one ever plans to lose their independence, so I hope you're getting the idea of just how important it is to KEEP your power source intact throughout your life, no matter your age.

Your body is designed to function in response to the physical stresses placed upon it. No physical stress in daily life equals loss of physical function. Muscles lose size and strength. Weakness ensues. Fatigue then comes from the simplest of activities.

And what happens when you go somewhere that's NOT designed to require NO physical activity on your part? What happens when you visit a grandchild and there are stairs to enter their home?

Want some good news? You're never too old to get stronger, and staying in shape is not that challenging. I just taught a live class the day before writing these words where most of the peeps in the class are in their 70s. We did 90 squats in that class in just seven and a half minutes! It wasn't a rush; we just went through five different arm motions as we squatted using three different foot positions with each of the arm motions. It was fabulous and everyone LOVED it!

Yes, there were those who needed to modify, maybe hold on and not go down as low or do as many reps, but most did the entire move and they were ALL smiling when we were done. No chair workouts for this group!

Remember Marge? Her left ankle was keeping her hips from doing what they needed to do during gait. This caused her right knee to compensate, which aggravated and irritated the knee structures, causing pain.

Conventional treatment may have included doing knee extensions to "strengthen" her knee. Unfortunately, these types of exercises often cause more harm than good because they create a lot of shear force in the knee structures.4 That exercise would've never restored the real culprit, impaired ankle function.

Over just a couple of weeks, Marge's ankle function radically improved, and she could now walk without knee pain. And guess what? I didn't wave a magic wand over her arthritis! That imaging report of OA had nothing to do with the reason she was experiencing pain. I have seen this kind of thing occur countless times while training people to resolve pain.

So, I hope I've convinced you to keep your stairs so you can stay stronger as you age. I repeat, no one ever plans to lose their independence so please plan to NOT lose the stairs!

CHAPTER 8

Shrinking, Humps, and "Turkey Neck," Aaarrrggghhh!

MYTH: Everyone gets shorter as they age.

Grimacing with determination, *Sister Joan pushed her head back toward the wall as far as she could. Disappointment replaced the grimace as I informed her the distance between the back of her head and the wall was 4.5 inches. Sister Joan was in her 90s and wanted to know what she could do to improve her posture during her time in therapy.*

She had an interesting childhood as her parents chose health care through an osteopath (this was in the 1920s) who often addressed issues with manual techniques when appropriate. Sister Joan was looking for anything she could do that perhaps she would have been taught by her family's osteopath. She was highly motivated to improve her posture and worked diligently to that end. I'll share what her head posture measured during our last session after you become more informed about why so many appear to "shrink" as they age.

Have you lost height? Are you inches shorter than you were in your younger years? Guess what? Losing height is NOT a normal part of aging. You may be talking out loud right now while reading this, saying, *"You don't know what you're talking about. Everyone gets shorter as they age!"*

Although many people do, in fact, lose height in their later years, it's NOT a *normal* process of aging. It may be *common*, but that doesn't make it *normal.*

A whole lot of folks have cardiovascular disease because it's common in the Western world. That doesn't make it normal. Disease is NOT normal. It is literally defined as *abnormal* functioning. So, getting shorter as you age is common, not normal.

Now that we've cleared that up, let's talk about why it happens and what you can do about it. There are basically three causes of diminishing height. Let's begin with what's commonly known first and go from there.

Posture

No one wants to hunch forward or grow shorter (isn't that an oxymoron?) as they age. Often the sole reason someone loses height is because of poor posture. It's not that their bones have shrunk. It's because their head is forward, which causes them to lose height when measured. Test this yourself. Try standing up straight and then slouch with your head dropping down and forward. You will see quite a difference in your height when measured in one position and then the other.

Let's begin at the beginning, so to speak. What happens with your posture after you're born?

At birth, your spine is more like a C curve. As you lift your head and learn to move, you develop what are called secondary curves. You begin to curve in (lordosis) at your neck and lower back. Your spine keeps the curve out (kyphosis) at your ribs and your pelvis. These natural meant-to-be-there curves allow your spine to be much stronger than if it were straight. The curves distribute and absorb stress much like the delicate-looking curved legs of an antique chair. The chair doesn't look like it could hold a 200-pound person, but it does because of the curves.

Spinal curves also provide flexibility and balance. Unfortunately, many people develop an imbalance in one or more of these curves. The curves at the low back and neck may flatten somewhat (decreased lordosis) or the curves at the trunk and pelvis may increase (hyper kyphosis). Of course, the opposite can happen as well. Imbalances can lead to pain and movement deficits; even respiration and digestion are compromised with an extreme kyphosis in the trunk.

Two of the most common postural imbalances are increased thoracic kyphosis (hunched upper back) or increased lumbar lordosis (swayed lower back). A forward head posture also creates a restriction at the base of the skull as your head tilts up to look forward, so you aren't looking at the ground. These things develop over time as other areas of the spine respond to create balance.

As in so many topics around health, there is much debate regarding posture and pain, and experts don't always agree. Go figure! It's been my experience that the more forward someone's head is, the more likely they are to have neck pain, headaches, shoulder pain, low back pain, and more, including poor balance.

It's simple physics. The longer the lever arm the more stress occurs. If you hold a 5 pound weight in your hand against your body, it feels like 5 pounds. Now hold your arm straight out from your body and 5 pounds feels more like 10 pounds or even 20 pounds.

Your head weighs on average about 12–15 pounds, depending on how smart you are. Just kidding! When your head shifts forward the stress to your muscles increases incrementally. One inch forward creates up to 20 pounds of pressure, two inches equals 30 pounds of pressure, and so on. Your neck muscles easily handle 12–15 pounds, not 30, 40, or even 50 pounds of pressure. This increased pressure leads to pain and dysfunction!

Why does the head go forward? It's kind of an "it depends on …" answer. Some people spend their lives sitting at a desk leaning forward or sitting behind the wheel of a taxi, bus, or 18-wheeler with their arms and head forward. After eight hours or more per day for decades, standing up straight becomes next to impossible. The muscles in the front of the body "lock short" and the person bends forward.

A lot of this occurs in the front hip muscles, which attach to the lumbar spine. This is why many people feel lower back pain upon standing after prolonged sitting. The front hip muscles pull on the lower back.

Standing without straightening up completely also keeps the head forward, and now gravity (that physics law nobody ever thinks about unless they're falling) plays a role in pulling the head down toward the ground. Those who spend their lives in a job that requires standing can also end up with a forward head. Jobs like being a cashier or a line cook require looking down all day, every day. What I find fascinating is not ALL people in these positions end up with severe posture issues. Many do, yet some don't. Hmmm ...

It's not uncommon to see people develop increased curves in their upper back. Technically this is termed hyper kyphosis with a Cobb angle of more than 40 degrees. It's also commonly called Dowager's Hump, humpback, round back, or hunchback. From ages 20 to 40, the kyphosis angle averages between 20 and 29 degrees; however, it can begin to increase significantly in both men and women after 40 years of age to as high as 52 degrees. Research reports varying incidences of hyper kyphosis, from 20 to 40 percent within both genders.[1] Aside from personal appearance, there are typical symptoms related to this issue, including back pain (mild to severe), inability to stand straight up that worsens as the day passes, and fatigue (mild to severe).

It's tiring to fight falling forward all day long! As this curvature progresses, it can lead to serious health issues such as difficulty breathing due to lung compression and even loss of appetite. All those inner organs are not happy with this posture!

There are three medical terms for kyphosis:

- Degenerative kyphosis occurs when the discs and vertebrae in the spine degenerate.
- Postural kyphosis occurs due to weak postural muscles and spinal changes.
- Iatrogenic kyphosis happens from medical intervention. Yes, medical treatment can cause kyphosis. Post-laminectomy kyphosis is the most common type of iatrogenic kyphosis, which can develop after spinal decompression surgery.

Now let's look at an issue that creates a lot of fear.

Compression Fractures

When vertebrae become weak and porous, they're prone to fracture, and usually this injury occurs in the anterior portion of the vertebrae (front), which then collapses. The posterior or back portion remains intact, which then creates a wedge shape that tips the spine forward. Of course, any of you who have taken my Nourish Your Body for Life classes or Women's Health Workshops know what leads to osteoporosis and, hopefully, are eating and exercising in a way that protects your bones. If you've not taken those courses, please read chapters 9 and 10.

You read earlier that osteoporosis is technically a risk factor for experiencing a fracture. Osteopenia is a risk factor for developing osteoporosis. So, osteopenia is a risk factor for a risk factor. You can very well live the rest of your life with no problems with a risk factor. It's your choices that make a difference. Shouldn't they be *informed* choices?

Why does this terminology about risk factors matter? I've seen women literally stop exercising, taking walks, or doing ANYTHING physical for fear of breaking something once they get this diagnosis. Ouch! This *fear* can literally snowball women into weakness, frailty, and bone loss due to lack of movement. Talk about perpetuating the absolute wrong thing in life because of a risk factor!!!

My goal here is to inform you of facts that matter in day-to-day life so you can make better decisions with improved outcomes. My passion is to erase fear and why it happens around this topic.

Fear is never a good strategy when making important health care decisions. I remember how terrified my mother was when she was told her spine was "degenerating" due to this diagnosis. She literally thought she was in grave danger of her spine disintegrating and that becoming an invalid in a wheelchair was in her future!

No one makes good decisions when gripped with fear. Generally, people (mostly women) are consistently warned they don't want to break a hip and end up in a nursing home, and look how many die within a year of breaking a hip. This is often the rationale used by well meaning health care providers when prescribing osteoporosis medications.

The practice of instilling fear infuriates me!! Mainly because it's not the whole truth and it serves no one well! I have worked in nursing home settings, and the broken hip is NOT the reason these people end up admitted in a nursing home or the reason they died within a year. Many who break a hip are *already debilitated,* with impaired function. They were already using walkers and had multiple serious health issues. The hip injury was simply the last straw that required complete physical dependence and care.

The *whole truth* is that multiple health issues are why many die within a year of a broken hip. It's NOT because of a broken hip. I repeat, it's NOT the broken hip. It's their physical and medical status PRIOR to a broken hip that leads to these heartbreaking statistics. The TRUTH is many of these injured folks were at the end of their lives already and they would have likely passed within a year even if they hadn't broken their hip.

This really changes the perspective, doesn't it?

I saw many, many people experience a broken hip, enter the nursing home for rehab, recover and return home to their prior level of independence ONLY if they were independent before their injury. The most important factor determining their outcome was their physical function and level of health PRIOR to the injury.

I'll never forget one woman in her 80s who had slipped from a ladder while she was cleaning snow off her roof! She was strong and relatively healthy when she had her accident. This woman recovered quickly and returned home completely independent! She also shared she would be back on a ladder if need be …

Yes, there are people who experience fractures due to poor bone health. My goal is to inform you of why this happens and the steps you can take that matter most, without fear influencing your decision making. Facts about osteoporosis are provided in several chapters to cover multiple areas such as medical testing, medical treatments, dietary factors, lifestyle choices, and exercise.

Degenerative disc disease (DDD) is another reason people lose height. DDD is not because of gravity, compression, or old age. It's been studied extensively by Dr. Leena Kauppila and can be seen whenever impaired blood supply occurs to the spine. I covered what causes impaired blood supply in chapter 3, remember?

Let's get back to posture. You may be surprised at what I'm about to tell you, but there's no such thing as perfect posture.

Surprised?! Ideal posture is just an "idea," and no one actually has it. It's stated as ideal because everything is aligned to allow for joints to be relatively stress free at rest and highly unlikely to be irritated or injured by movement. Your posture is also how your body balances. If your body doesn't balance, you fall.

So, what's the goal if ideal posture is not attainable in real life? The goal is to get as close to it as possible. The further away from ideal posture your body resides, the more likely you are to experience chronic pain patterns, limited mobility, and balance issues.

The more imbalance and asymmetry your body demonstrates from poor posture, the more likely you'll have pain. There's also the whole forward-head thing pulling you into a kyphotic hump that no one wants as well as losing height as the years tick by.

I'll now provide some details about ideal posture and then talk about what can go awry, concluding with what you can do about it. Sound good?

Ideal Posture

Analyzing your posture is not only looking at your bones and how they align. True postural analysis is an assessment of the function of your motor system (bones, muscles, and ligaments) and your nervous and fascial system's control of your motor system.

To assess static standing posture, a plumb line is often used, showing specific points of the body where gravity "passes through." Ideal posture has a plumb line intersecting the ankle, knee, hip joint, center of gravity, shoulder, and ear.

When aligned well, your joints are relatively stress free at rest and unlikely to be irritated or injured by movement.

If you don't have a plumb line handy and want to assess posture, let me walk you through an assessment of your curves by lying down on your back with arms and legs extended and palms up. Close your eyes and notice how your body contacts the floor.

Ideal posture, when lying down, people notice:

- the center of the back of the skull resting comfortably on the floor (not looking up behind you)
- the lower ribs (just below the shoulder blades) bearing the weight of the torso
- the buttocks bearing the weight of the pelvis (no tailbone poking into the floor)
- both thighs bearing weight midway down (not floating)
- the calves bearing weight
- the heels bearing weight with the feet shaped like the letter V (not turned out resting on the ankle bones or straight up toward the ceiling)
- both sides of the body (right and left) feel evenly weighted as well as even in length (arms and legs)

How did you do with this assessment? Is your posture anywhere close to ideal? Keep reading to see what common asymmetries or imbalances are and finally what you can do about it.

Common imbalances people notice:

- the head resting as if you are looking up OR needing a pillow (or two)
- one or both shoulder blades poking into the floor
- the lower ribs (just below the shoulder blades) floating off the floor
- a big whaling arch in the mid back
- the tailbone poking into the floor
- one or both thighs floating off the floor
- one or both feet turned out and resting on the ankle bones OR pointed straight up
- one side of the body feels heavier
- one side of the body feels longer (one arm or one leg)

How many imbalances did you notice during your assessment?

You can take this a step further during your lying assessment and understand there are three places your body will exhibit imbalances the most: your shoulder girdle, your mid back, and your pelvis.

If your shoulder girdle is imbalanced, you may notice when you turn your head that there is pain or limited motion on one side (or both). Your lower ribs may be floating and not bearing weight.

If your pelvis is imbalanced, you may feel a big arch in your back, from your pelvis up to your ribs. That's a common issue that often leads to back, hip, shoulder, or neck pain. You may also notice a lot of weight on your tailbone and one or both of your thighs floating.

The last big issue contributing to chronic pain or mobility/balance issues is if you notice one side of your body feels heavier or longer. This is impaired communication and inefficiency in your body.

Your posture exposes adaptations and compensations accumulated from injuries, habits, and medical issues that you've experienced during your lifetime. It's NOT a result of the process of aging! I've been the same height since reaching adulthood. My head is over my shoulders where it belongs, and I turn 66 on my next birthday.

Your body learns to adapt and compensate to allow you to balance and function as effectively as possible; yet it can only compensate so far and then things begin to break down. This happens to young people too. I've worked with people of all ages whose bodies have been compensating for things that went awry somewhere along the way. Have you seen the posture of young people nowadays because of constant cellphone usage?

What to Do About It

So, you noticed at least one or two imbalances (maybe even four or five) and you want to do something about it! There's more than one way, but I expect you've learned by now attempting to remember to stand up straight isn't one of them. This is because other thoughts need your time and attention throughout the day.

What you CAN do is perform movements designed to address the common culprits of the imbalances OR you can learn to self-treat your fascial system OR you can do both, which I highly recommend.

The right movements performed repetitively promote success in improving common imbalances. They MUST be performed without pain and without the need to compensate due to pain or impaired balance. This means minimizing the movements or holding on for support while doing them and building on your success.

Success means NO pain or struggle to keep your balance. Your brain will cheat if you feel pain repetitively. Your brain will also cheat if your balance is at risk. You won't know you're cheating, and you will literally be training in dysfunction and compensatory patterns. That is NOT success.

Because movements (especially with modifications) are not well taught when written, I have videos on my YouTube channel on posture. I host free events online regularly that include posture education and training. Check the Resources. If you're determined to age really stinkin' well, like I am, you might want to check those out. Just a thought ...

To finish Sister Joan's story, I'm thrilled to tell you she was able to improve her forward head posture from 4.5 inches away from the wall to just 1.5 inches. She improved by 3 inches in just a few weeks, and she was in her 90s! I'm betting she continued to improve, but she was discharged as the other reason she was receiving therapy had resolved, so I can't say for sure.

PART 3

Methods and Options Your Doctor (or PT or Chiropractor) May Not Know About

Part 3 is where the rubber meets the road. This is information aimed to empower you to make changes that can transform your future. This is the part many will go to first. If that's the case, PLEASE read the first two parts ASAP. Why is this important?

Doing the Homework Makes All the Difference

In my profession, I saw two types of patients: those that didn't do their homework and those that did.

Those that didn't do their homework saw little progress and continued to complain about the reason they were coming to the clinic.

Those that did their homework saw success often and "graduated" from PT with flying colors. They were the ones who wrote thank-you cards that we put up on the wall so others could be encouraged.

Why were some compliant and some not? A lack of understanding versus a full understanding was what made the difference. Understanding why they were told to do what they needed to do to get better made for a higher level of compliance and much more success.

Example: If you understand working to improve strength in your hips will help to resolve chronic back pain, you'll do your hip exercises. If you don't understand this, you'll think why bother. This won't work. It's a waste of my time. She didn't even give me any exercises for my back. You may not even bother to return to the clinic.

Increased Compliance

Part 3 is more about the homework needed to change things. Parts 1 and 2 are more about understanding why the homework is necessary. This will greatly improve your compliance with doing the work.

Make sense?

CHAPTER 9

Nourish to Age Without Dementia and More

MYTH: Alzheimer's just happens.

In his book *Dying Young,* Dr. Lester Packer writes, "More than 70% of Americans will die prematurely from diseases caused by or compounded by deficiencies of the antioxidant network."

In other words, at least seven out of ten Americans die before their time due to not eating enough fruits and vegetables. There really is something to this thing about eating plant foods, especially when it comes to healthy aging, including your brain!

I saw the difference in my patients based on the food in their kitchens. Those who ate fruits and vegetables exhibited a much higher quality of life overall than those whose counters were covered with sweets and junk foods. The latter were always in need of assistive devices and dependent on others for day-to-day function.

Margaret Mead said, *"It is easier to change a man's religion than to change his diet."* I don't think this is true for all people. How about you?

Brain Health and Aging

No one EVER wants to lose their memory. Dementia affects more than 55 million people worldwide, with 10 million people being diagnosed each year.[1] Of them, 60 to 70 percent have Alzheimer's Disease (AD), which is a type of dementia. In the U.S., AD affects almost 6 million people, adversely impacting their families and communities, not to mention the human misery experienced by all involved.

Providing more dismal statistics, dementia is the seventh leading cause of death among all diseases and the third leading cause of death after cancer and heart disease in certain age groups. The World Health Organization predicts the number of people with dementia will rise to 78 million by 2030 and 139 million by 2050. The more people become informed of the risk factors, the more this will cause the general population to make different choices with improved outcomes. The ultimate goal of this book is to change what is commonly seen!

Let me share a positive statement written on the WHO website.

"Although age is the strongest known risk factor for dementia, it is ***not an inevitable consequence of biological aging****"* (emphasis mine).

The lifetime risk for Alzheimer's at age 45 is one in five for women and one in ten for men. *Doesn't this mean four out of five women and nine out of ten men WON'T get Alzheimer's?!*

Dementia doesn't have to happen! We're not at the mercy of fate, luck of the draw, or genetics. We can reduce our risk of cognitive decline and dementia by:

- being physically active
- not smoking
- avoiding harmful use of alcohol
- controlling our weight
- eating a healthy diet
- maintaining healthy blood pressure, cholesterol, and blood sugar levels

I'm going to focus on food in this chapter. So, the question is this: *"Is diet seen to influence your risk of dementia?"*

Dr. Christopher Weber, director of global science initiatives at the Alzheimer's Association, states: *"Research looking at the relationship between diet and cognition is well-established. There is strong evidence to suggest that what is good for the heart is good for the head, and we know a healthy diet is good for the heart."*

Unfortunately, differences of opinion abound when the topic of what constitutes a healthy diet comes up, even for the heart. My father was provided a "heart healthy" diet in the hospital when he underwent a stent procedure in his early 80s after having two heart attacks in a 24-hour period. He was provided meats covered in gravy, chicken or tuna salad sandwiches with an extra packet of mayo, and other jaw-dropping food choices labeled heart healthy on his meal ticket. That's another topic.

Now I want to share what studies show, and then we'll conclude with what's shown to have the most impact on healthy aging overall.

Have you heard of the MIND Diet? It's the Mediterranean Intervention for Neurodegenerative Delay.[2] Creative acronym, don't you think?

It's like the Mediterranean diet, focusing on green leafy vegetables, other vegetables, nuts, berries, beans, whole grains, seafood, poultry, olive oil, and wine. Of course, if it has the word Mediterranean in it, olive oil and wine are always part of the equation. The truth is plants protect our circulation, not oils, which you learned earlier.

The study highlights the importance of foods and nutrients having an association with dementia prevention, with those showing the highest scores equivalent of being seven and a half years younger in age. Diet is significantly associated with each cognitive domain, particularly episodic memory, semantic memory, and perceptual speed:[3]

- **Episodic**: memory of specific events unique to each person, influenced by semantic memory
- **Semantic:** general world knowledge accumulated throughout lifetime
- **Perceptual speed:** ability to accurately (and completely) compare letters, numbers, objects, pictures, or patterns when tested

Studies also report that processed food may increase the risk of dementia. Typically, they're high in refined carbohydrates[4] (sugar and white flour). Processed meats such as sausage, salami, and bacon were seen to increase the risk of all dementias by 44 percent and AD by 52 percent.[5]

A healthy diet was one of the six habits linked to a lower risk of dementia and a slower rate of memory decline. In total, 29,072 participants were followed for ten years to collect this data.[6] Additional risk factors reported by the WHO are seen to coincide with this list as they include depression, social isolation, and cognitive inactivity. I won't get off on a tangent, but did you know depression is positively impacted by exercise? Read *Spark* by Dr. John Ratey to learn more.

These are the six habits linked to cognitive and memory health:

- Healthy diet
- Exercising mind
- Regular physical exercise
- Active social contact
- No alcohol
- No smoking

It's no surprise to me that daily intake of plant foods was seen to have the strongest effect on slowing memory decline. Notice the NO alcohol? What happened to the wine? Let's divert from food for a moment because the alcohol question is an important one if you enjoy a glass of wine with a special meal or a cold beer on a hot summer day.

The challenges to studying this detail are numerous, including the fact alcohol consumption is self-reported. People are notorious for under-reporting so-called bad habits and over-reporting so-called good habits. Each study measured amounts differently and what constituted light versus moderate versus heavy drinking differed, challenging clear conclusions. Add the fact those put into the non-drinking group may have quit drinking due to health concerns from previous heavy drinking and you can see how difficult this is to decipher clearly and tease out important variables for an accurate picture.

In a study of centenarians, only 11 percent of the males and 22 percent of the females reported *never* consuming alcohol.[7] This means *never* having alcohol may not be required to live a long quality life.

It's disappointing this particular study looked at pretty much everything in their lives (medical/dental history, occupation, education, genealogy, and so on) except what they ate!

However, they did look at 300 centenarians. Next to their retained cognitive functioning, the large majority had moderate-good hearing and vision abilities, were independently mobile, enjoyed independence in activities of daily living, and had no or few symptoms of depression. Yes, you CAN age with joy!

Circulatory Health and Aging

Not having a heart attack or a stroke certainly improves your odds of having a quality life that doesn't end earlier than it should. Let's look at some data about how food impacts these issues.

The first sign of cardiovascular disease (CVD) is often sudden death from a heart attack or a stroke. CVD is known to be the leading cause of death in the U.S., with someone dying every 33 seconds from a heart attack and every three minutes from a stroke.[8] The American Heart Association has funded more than $5 billion in research since 1949. It would appear they're not having a very good return on their investment.

Reported risk factors:

- Smoking
- Physical inactivity
- Nutrition
- Excess weight
- Cholesterol
- Sleep
- Diabetes
- High blood pressure

Leading dietary risk factors were high sodium intake, low whole grain intake, and low legume intake.

When nutrition is reported in these main sites, there's no mention of saturated fats, oils, and other foods that we know injure the endothelial cells that line all your blood vessels, leading to increased blood pressure, plaques, heart attacks, and strokes.

Dr. David Blankenhorn compared effects of different types of fats on the growth of atherosclerotic lesions inside the coronary arteries by studying the results of angiograms taken one year apart.[9] The study showed all three types of fat, saturated animal fat, monounsaturated (olive oil), and polyunsaturated (EFA), were linked with a significant increase in new atherosclerotic lesions. Most importantly, the growth of these lesions did not stop when polyunsaturated fats and monounsaturated fats were substituted for saturated fats.

Now, to stomp again on a subject that may cause you to shut this book and yell out loud … wait for it …

The University of Maryland did a study on the effect of eating bread dipped in *olive oil* and reported a reduced dilation in the brachial artery, indicating injury to the endothelial cells that line the blood vessels and impairment of nitric oxide production.[10]

That's how the popular drug, Viagra, works. It increases the production of nitric oxide. I heard an expert present *Erectile Dysfunction (ED), the Canary in the Coal Mine*, which showed impaired circulation is the culprit behind ED and may be the first warning sign a man has CVD.

Here's more in case you're not yet convinced oils aren't your friend. It's reported that both omega-3 and omega-6 contribute to the development of plaques, damaging the arteries.[11,12]

Last one before we move on. The *British Medical Journal* analyzed the results of 48 randomized controlled trials and 41 cohort studies. That means 89 studies showed no evidence of reduced risk of cardiovascular events or mortality from taking omega-3.[13]

So, plants, not plant oils, are what we need to consume to protect our circulation.

Bone Health and Aging

Here's the nitty-gritty on how food directly impacts bone health and why the "Calcium Paradox" exists.[14–17]

Your blood pH must stay between 7.35 and 7.45 because even minor fluctuations can adversely affect many organs and cause serious health issues, even convulsions and death.

Your body has three major buffering systems to prevent dietary and metabolic acids from shifting the pH outside the narrow range needed to maintain life:

1. Kidneys: eliminate excess hydrogen ions (H+/acids) through the urine
2. Lungs: eliminate carbon dioxide
3. Buffer salts: stored reserves of alkaline minerals can be drawn upon to neutralize acids

These buffering systems, which neutralize and remove excess acids, are always at work maintaining pH balance in the body.

Eating large amounts of high-acid-load foods like animal protein, including cheese/dairy, combined with the challenge for your kidneys to excrete waste byproducts from these foods, causes a need for buffering agents. Where are these stored? In your bones.

Excess acid consumption not only depletes buffer salt reserves, but also puts a strain on the kidneys and the lungs. If the kidneys or lungs are impaired in any way, acids build up in the body. When the body's ability to neutralize excess acids is impaired, acidosis can occur.

Protein contains nitrogen and the need to metabolize excess nitrogen leads to creating acid byproducts, specifically uric and sulfuric acids.

This byproduct must be neutralized prior to excretion to maintain life-sustaining blood pH levels. This is why increased dairy product intake is seen to lead to higher fracture risk—ergo, the Calcium Paradox.

According to the National Academy of Sciences, 1 gram of protein increases calcium excretion in the urine by 1 to 1.5 milligrams. A 4-ounce serving of meat has 20 grams of protein, which results in 30 milligrams of calcium in the urine.

Reducing animal protein consumption (and eliminating dairy foods) results in reduced calcium excretion. Out of 18 published studies, 14 (around 80 percent) support low-acid eating as a means to preserve bones or improve bone health.[18]

High phosphorus intake also causes your parathyroid gland to draw calcium from your bones to match the phosphorus levels. Meat and milk are high in both phosphorus and protein. Phosphates are also added to soft drinks and refined and processed foods. The RDA for adults is 700 milligrams/day, and the Standard American Diet has two to four times more phosphorus than calcium.

Animal foods contain ten to twenty times as much phosphorus as calcium, and soft drinks have as much as 500 milligrams of phosphorus per serving. Fruits and vegetables, on the other hand, don't contain high levels of these acid-forming amino acids, and instead have a predominantly alkaline-forming mineral composition.

In the *Postgraduate Medical Journal*,[19] a critical review states:

> Many official bodies give advice on desirable intakes of calcium but there is no clear evidence of a calcium deficiency disease in otherwise normal people that has ever been shown. In Western countries the usual calcium intake is of the order of 800-1000 mg/day. In many developing countries figures of 300-500 mg/day are found. There is no evidence that people with such a low intake have any problems with bones or teeth. It seems likely that normal people can adapt to have a normal calcium balance on calcium intakes as low as 150-200 mg/day and that this adaptation is sufficient even in pregnancy and lactation. Inappropriate concern about calcium intake may divert attention and resources from more important nutritional problems.

The U.S. RDA for calcium is set above human requirements to provide a wide margin of safety for the majority of Americans. It's not due to evidence-based needs. Taking calcium supplements results in more cardiovascular events than reductions in the fractures they are supposed to prevent.

A 30 percent increase in risk of heart attack is reported in scientific data with 500 mg calcium per day. People consuming a diet with lower calcium intake don't develop health issues or impaired bone development as a result. A high-calcium diet results in lower calcium absorption, and a lower calcium intake results in higher calcium absorption.[20,21]

There've been some recent mentions about the source of the buffering agents the body uses to neutralize acid load being in the food itself. I've read some of these studies and am not convinced the conclusions are accurate. Too many details to cover here. Ergo, the Resources section.

Muscle Health and Aging

This is a subject that has prioritized protein intake since the ancient Olympics in 776 B.C. Scientists and athletes have debated about the perfect diet for athletes, but what about someone who just wants to be fit and healthy, not win a Gold Medal?

Countless articles state older people need to increase their protein intake so they don't lose muscle. This is inaccurate. I did a deep dive into the data surrounding sarcopenia, otherwise known as age-related lean muscle mass. The studies are not conclusive that it's due to age alone, but more due to inactivity and lack of exercise. It's a **time**-related issue of being sedentary and not an **age**-related issue.

As far as food and muscles are concerned, nobody builds muscle in the kitchen. It ALWAYS requires physical training; however, how you fuel your body can enhance your results.

Did you know building muscle is dependent on the number of calories you consume to provide the energy needed for strength training? If you're struggling to build muscle, you may not be consuming enough calories, not lacking protein. Studies show it's the amount of *carbohydrates* you consume that impact muscle growth. Complex carbohydrates also decrease delayed-onset muscle soreness.

Consuming too little carbohydrate and focusing on protein intake leads to protein being burned for *fuel* and not used for muscle *growth.* Fifteen percent of calories from protein is more than adequate based on the assumption that calorie intake is adequate. Vegetables have protein. Plant protein is just as good as animal protein. The whole complete versus incomplete protein topic is misleading. A whole-food plant-based diet is not lacking in protein.

The Institute of Medicine reports that *"no additional dietary protein is suggested for healthy adults undertaking resistance or endurance exercise."*[22]

Hydration is equally important as muscles are 78 percent water. If you're even mildly dehydrated, you'll struggle to grow muscle.[23,24] Muscles cramp when they don't have enough water. Ouch!

Disc Health and Aging

Remember Dr. Leena Kauppila, who spent decades looking at the impact impaired circulation has on the health of your spine, specifically the discs and the vertebrae? I introduced you to her in chapter 3. She published numerous studies showing impaired circulation to the lumbar arteries is seen to increase the occurrence of degenerative disc disease.[25,26]

If you have degenerative disc disease, it's not because of gravity, compression, or old age. It's due to impaired circulation. Because what you eat either injures or protects your circulation, this means you can impact your disc health through diet. Yay!

Joint Health and Aging

Remember, the Stanford University School of Medicine did a study to determine the cause of joint damage.[27] It's not due to old age, wear and tear, or compression. It's due to chronic inflammation.

Food and chronic inflammation data is profound. I can share story after story of people who saw joint pain diminish, even disappear, after changing their diet. But although those testimonials may impress people, they don't validate that the average person would experience the same result if they changed their diet. That type of validation requires clinical studies.

Hopefully, you read chapter 3, so you have more details on other things reported about a chronic inflammatory state such as arachidonic acid overload from too many animal foods consumed and fat cell promotion of inflammatory chemicals when carrying excess weight. Here, I want to share what you can ADD to your diet that enhances positive changes.

There are countless studies showing direct changes in blood biomarkers for inflammation by changing food intake. Studies include whole grains,[28] cruciferous vegetables,[29] and more. There are also many studies that show chronic pain correlates with how many vegetables are consumed daily.[30] Even the risk of developing knee OA is shown to be reduced by over 60 percent by an increased intake of fiber.[31] Fiber is only found in plants.

I could write an entire book on this one topic, but I'm hoping you get the idea.

Yes, what you put in your mouth matters not only for your overall health, but also impacts brain, heart, bone, and joint health. A low-fat, whole-food, plant-based way of eating is a strategy that promotes profound health in the human body.

You may need some guidance to achieve success if this is new to you. According to a 2012 study, more than 50 percent of Americans (that were polled) felt that doing their taxes is easier than figuring out how to eat healthy. This is most likely due to all the conflicting information prevalent in our world. Please know a healthy diet is not brain surgery. It can be simple once you learn the basics.

Resources has some simple, quick recipes that received rave reviews from the Nourish Away Pain classes taught at a local community college. Real food for real people, not just salads.

CHAPTER 10

Exercise Your Body the Right Way for Pain-Free Strength and Healthy Bones

MYTH: You can't grow muscles when you're old.

I want to remind you of Question #2 from chapter 1. What have you heard about muscle growth and aging? Everywhere you look, you'll read articles spouting how age-related muscle loss is normal. This is not accurate, as you read earlier. It's not my opinion or ignorance of the truth.

Yes, you can find lots of information spouting physiological reasons why older people lose muscle more easily than younger people. Reasons like "anabolic resistance," which means the body doesn't respond as well to the signals that normally cause muscles to grow bigger and stronger since anabolism is the building up of muscle.

Catabolism is the breaking down of things, and a "catabolic crisis," which is muscle loss in size and strength, is much more likely to occur if a perfect storm happens.

What's a perfect storm?

A perfect storm is when things like the world lockdown occurred, poor sleep quality due to extreme stress from fear and worry was common, and a huge potential for being bedridden due to illness ensued.

How is this due to age?! So many studies regurgitate the same old, same old ... *"Muscle loss is an inevitable fact of aging."* NO! More and more well done studies are showing those who perform weightlifting exercises *don't lose muscle.* It's a lack of *exercise,* not a fact of *age.*

A 2023 study reported that 73-year-old powerlifters and weightlifters maintained Type II muscle fiber distribution similar to 25 younger adults.[1] Type II muscle fiber provides strength and power. Lifelong endurance athletes, like runners, didn't show the same results. They showed more effect of muscle "aging" than powerlifters. Endurance activities require more Type I muscle fiber, which provides what's needed for runners.

Weight training is truly what's needed to stay strong OR to regain strength if lost.

You read in the last chapter that high-protein diets are not required to build and maintain muscle. As stated earlier, we could build muscle in the kitchen and never need to exercise if that were true.

Aging and Muscle Growth

You've read how loss of muscle (sarcopenia) is time-related, but this means related to the amount of time that someone does NOT exercise and lives a very sedentary life. It's NOT due to age, as many people in their 90s and beyond have shown they can get stronger.

Let me tell you about some folks who proved this in real life.

At the age of 91, Sy Perlis broke a world record in 2013 by bench pressing 187.2 pounds! I shared this at a conference and asked the audience, including many younger men present, if anyone there could bench press that amount of weight. No one raised their hand.

The best part? Sy didn't start weight training until he was 60 and he didn't start competing until his 80s!

Julia Hawkins, at 105 years old, ran 100 meters in 63 seconds.

It's never too late to start. This was proven by an entire group of older women in the Bill Beekley Academy of Powerlifting.

Bonnie Thurston, at the age of 78 has a current goal of being able to deadlift 200 pounds! Seven years prior to this goal, Bonnie was diagnosed with osteoporosis. She found and joined a powerlifting group for older women where they deadlift, bench press, and pull weighted sleds.

Edith Murway-Traina, still powerlifting at 99 years old, started weight training at 91! I watched her deadlift almost 100 pounds! They're all trained by expert Bill Beekley, who has trained powerlifters for decades, preventing their risk of injury.

I loved Edith's statements in the CBS news video feed: *"I've always had muscles. I just had to learn to use them … The more you move, the more exercise you get, the more your body responds."*

Resources provides links to view these ordinary seniors who demonstrate extraordinarily uncommon aging. Notice I didn't say abnormal?

Training to Grow Muscle at Any Age

There are different types of muscle fibers: Type I and Type II.

Type I is also known as slow-twitch muscle fibers or red fibers. They provide what is needed in low-resistance, high-repetition, or long-duration, low-intensity training. Consider aerobic activities like marathons and triathlons. These muscle fibers also provide stabilization and postural control needed whenever you're upright.

Type II is also known as fast-twitch muscle fibers or white fibers. They provide what's needed for greater and quicker force. Type II can also be broken down into Type IIb and Type IIa. Type IIb produces the most force, but it's inefficient and fatigues quickly. Type IIa is a mix of Type I and Type IIb so it fatigues slower. Type II fibers support power activities like bench pressing and squats. In real life, you use these muscles to get something heavy out of the trunk of your car.

All muscles are a mix of fast-twitch and slow-twitch muscle fibers. Whether you have more of one than the other depends on your activity level. Some say age is a factor, but I hope you've learned by now this is inaccurate. It's a *time* factor based on consistent activity levels.

*Non*athletic individuals have close to a 50/50 balance of fiber types. Highly skilled, top-performing athletes have a higher ratio of one to the other depending on their sport. Power athletes have a higher ratio of fast-twitch fibers (70 to 75 percent). Endurance athletes have more slow-twitch fibers (70 to 80 percent).

Want good news? You can modify your fiber types through exercise. Resistance training increases the size of both Type I and Type II muscle fibers. Greater growth occurs in Type II fibers and increases both actin and myosin filaments. This results in an increased ability to generate force. That means more strength when you need it.

Here's where I must share a commonly parroted statement that causes me to feel anger. It's the "no pain, no gain" statement. So many have been harmed, even injured, because of misunderstanding this statement. Let's clarify how you can protect yourself from potential injury.

No pain, no gain is a way to describe delayed onset muscle soreness (DOMS)[2] that occurs after exercise. It doesn't mean it's okay for the exercise to hurt. DOMS is most often due to a new activity or increasing the intensity or duration of a well known activity, which causes micro-tears in muscles. This leads to a presence of cytokines, neutrophils, monocytes, and macrophages and results in production of reactive oxygen species (ROS) and reduced use of ATP.

In plain English, this means the muscle has been injured and needs to repair. The repair process typically leads to bigger and stronger muscles, thus the no pain, no gain statement. This soreness peaks 24 to 48 hours after exercise and normally lasts one to two days, at most four days. While sore, you'll notice a lower range of motion, reduced strength, and a lower performance level.

Caution! Countless supplements tout they'll reduce DOMS, yet there is little evidence to support that claim and not much effect. What's been seen to impact DOMS in a positive way is consuming sufficient calories, complex carbohydrate intake, and good hydration habits. Hopefully, you read the last chapter and learned all about that.

So, how does a skeletal muscle grow bigger? For those who enjoy details, there are two types of muscular hypertrophy:

1. Myofibrillar: growth of muscle contraction parts that increases strength and speed.
2. Sarcoplasmic: increased muscle glycogen storage, which increases energy storage and endurance.

Skeletal muscle contraction initiation and execution details are quite complex. In addition to chemical changes, there are also specialized receptors on the surface of muscle cells that detect when you move a muscle, generate force, or otherwise alter the biochemical machinery within a muscle.

In a healthy young person, when these systems detect muscle movement, they turn on a number of specialized chemical pathways within the muscle. These pathways in turn trigger the production of more proteins that get incorporated into the muscle fibers and cause the muscle to increase in size.

These cellular pathways also turn on genes that code for specific proteins in cells that make up the muscles' contracting machinery. This activation of gene expression is a longer-term process, with genes being turned on or off for several hours after a single session of resistance exercise.

The bottom-line effect of these many exercise-induced changes is to cause your muscles to get bigger. I want to point out it all began with muscle *contraction.* That doesn't happen without exercise, and resistance is required. It's not about eating more animal protein.

Pain and Exercise

I now want to share some important information, especially if you've not read my book, *Pain Culprits!* If you have pain that limits your ability to exercise, it just might be that your body requires some conditioning in three-plane function. Many struggle with exercise or lack results due to pain, not age.

If you have a knee that doesn't like squats and it's not "bone on bone," it just may be due to an impairment in your hip or ankle. Your knee is made up of the femur (hip to knee) and tibia/fibula (ankle to knee) so it's really your lower hip and upper ankle.

Many who needlessly suffer from knee pain have found relief when they address the real culprit behind the problem. Your knee is most often a victim.

What about lower back pain? That can often improve by ignoring the back and addressing hip or trunk function. Your low back is a torque converter between your hips and trunk. This means if your hip lacks function, your lower back is unable to transfer the torque created by your trunk up above when turning, so your lower back says "ouch." The flip side is if your trunk lacks function, your lower back is unable to transfer the torque created by your hips rotating below, so your lower back complains.

To keep this moving along, your shoulder is dependent on healthy pelvis, trunk, and shoulder blade function. Your rotator cuff has only four muscles. There are eighteen muscles directly impacting shoulder function, and the whole rest of the body indirectly impacts shoulder function. Shoulder pain is rarely due to rotator cuff issues!

My YouTube channel teaches details of how important full ankle mobility and stability are to the entire rest of your body when walking or doing any physical activity or sport. It's the Plantar Fasciitis playlist. You don't need to have PF to benefit from knowing how important ankle function is to all human movement.

I hope you're getting the idea. Everything is connected to everything else. So many are unable to exercise without pain but the body part complaining is often not the body part causing the problem. That's why treatment often fails.

Another important factor with exercise is to make sure it's authentic and used in real life. This means not isolating muscles because you don't do that when lifting something heavy out of the trunk of your car or squatting down to pick up a grandchild.

Many believe they must work specific muscles on specific days. Often, these exercises attempt to isolate a muscle. The problem is that this can't really be done. It's a physics thing. For every action, there's an equal and opposite reaction. When you exercise a hip, the other hip is always impacted. When you do a biceps curl, your body reacts with an equal and opposite force, or you wouldn't be able to lift the weight.

The hundreds of muscles in your body are designed to work as a team, helping each other to accomplish the task. When you attempt to isolate, you disrupt the team and put much-needed players on the bench. This leads to pain issues such as tendinopathy and tendonitis. I've seen many, many patients in the clinic with a diagnosis of tendonitis who went to the gym four or five days a week. The best part? These issues were best helped by performing authentic eccentric loading.[3]

Another thing I want to cover is if the movement itself is authentic. Is it a movement your body would normally do, whether in daily life or in a sports setting?

Can you tell me when you would ever stand and kick your foot toward your butt against resistance in repetition? Yes, hamstring curls strengthen your hamstrings, but often at the expense of another body part, like your knees, not being happy.

Your hamstrings work in the context of the activity you're doing. When you walk, your hamstrings assist knee extension (the opposite of bending) while controlling the leg that's swinging forward. All the resisted hamstring curls in the world won't improve gait because your hamstrings don't do that in gait.

If you look around at the gym, you'll notice many exercises that aren't authentic. If you wouldn't do that movement in real life, it's wise to not do it against resistance in repetition.

Bone Health and Exercise

Strong bones are made by weight bearing exercise. If you have osteoporosis, you must be careful to do the right things the right way. There's an extremely skilled and experienced physical therapist by the name of Sherri R. Betz, PT, DPT, GCS, NCPT.

She has spent her entire career working with women to improve their strength safely, despite poor bone health. Many learn to do a deadlift with 50 pounds safely! I highly recommend you seek out expert guidance to do the right things the right way.

The data? Yes, resistance training can improve bone density. Certain activities can maintain bone health as well. Exercising regularly reduces the rate of bone loss and conserves bone tissue, lowering the risk of fractures.

The National Osteoporosis Foundation suggests high- or low-impact, weight-bearing, and muscle-strengthening exercises to prevent osteoporosis. These include jumping, jogging, and aerobics as high-impact exercises as well as walking and step aerobics as lower impact exercises.[4]

Studies showed some improvements in bone density in some bones but not in others. One example is whole-body vibration studies showed no improvement in lumbar spine density, only hip and tibia (shin bone). Weight-bearing aerobic exercises and strength training were the overall winners for results.[5]

This means things like walking, stair climbing, jogging, volleyball, tennis and similar sports, Tai Chi, and dancing as well as weight training with free weights, tubing or bands, or one's own body weight.

You should know the following details:

- Isolated exercise (single bout training) provides a fleeting bone-building stimulation.
- Longer training (for example, five weeks) provides better stimulation.
- Aerobic exercise is particularly effective in the enzymatic activation of the osteoblasts (bone builders).

This means it's important to combine both aerobic and resistance exercises in bone-building protocols.

Another very important factor is to include stability and balance exercises. Preventing falls is key to preventing injury, and aging well requires no fear of falling when you step down from a curb.

The last thing I want to cover is the importance of conditioning your body in all three planes of motion. The reason you don't look like a robot when moving is because you move in three planes, not just one. Yet, we learned to exercise in just one plane most of the time.

The problem with this is when you go to do real-life things like lifting a heavy bag of garden mulch, you aren't only lifting in one plane. *Your body must be trained the way you use it in real life.* That's the way to radically reduce the risk of injury while improving strength.

Because teaching movement in written words lacks visually dynamic detail, I have free videos that teach you how to not only move and train in three planes, but also assess your three-plane function to determine your potential culprits if you have pain anywhere. Please check Resources.

In summary, when it comes to conditioning your body the right way for pain-free strength, healthy muscles, and strong bones, you must know the following:

- Everything's connected to everything else.
- You must train in three planes of motion.
- The movement must be authentic and not isolated.
- It's most valuable when done on your feet because that's how you live your life.

There are no magic pills that restore or maintain physical function. You must do the work.

CHAPTER 11

Four Simple, Immediate Strategies to Reverse Aging Now

MYTH: Nothing can be done at your age.

I really kind of want to title this chapter *The Raspberry!* You know, when you stick out your tongue and make noise?

It's about showing the world that aging doesn't have to be a loss of independence with pain in every movement, a decline into disposable underwear, and a shoebox of meds by your side.

I've thought long and hard about what information to provide in this chapter, believing this may be the first chapter you flip to out of curiosity or the need to begin now as time is of the essence in your current world.

Before we begin, I want to remind you there are no magic pills in life. There is no magic pill that makes you physically stronger. There is no magic pill that causes you to nourish your body better. There is no magic pill that puts you in the "healing and repair nervous system" mode and takes you out of the "run from the bear" mode.

There is no magic pill.

I know the media and advertisement world would love for us to believe there is one, so we rush out to buy when it's promoted, but please hear me. *Do you know what snake oil is?*

There are decisions and choices to make. Actions based on those decisions are then required for you to see the results you are seeking. Yes, you can apply strategies to improve your success by taking the necessary actions but, I repeat, there are no magic pills. Now that we've cleared that up …

Ready? Let's go!

Strategy #1: MOVEMENT

The most valuable strategy to begin right now is to move. I don't mean homes; I mean your body. Before you complain this is not aligned with the title that states simple, immediate strategies to reverse aging now, I beg to differ. Moving is simple. The world of gurus and medical experts have complicated things. AND I provide you with a video movement assessment and training class that keeps it simple, teaching you how to modify your movements due to pain or other limitations. Check Resources.

Teaching exercise in written form is destined to fail. Movement requires seeing the actual movement. Modifications can be multi-faceted, and no one is going to read three pages of instruction to perform an exercise. Most people will just look at the picture and try it. That's when potential pain or injury occurs.

No matter your starting point (remember Question #1 in chapter 1?) you can begin moving your body in a way that does not elicit pain and provides great benefit in many ways. "Motion is lotion."

How often have you seen someone who sits for a while and has trouble moving once they stand up? They got stiff, had trouble with the first few steps but, after a moment or two, they began to move more smoothly. I repeat. Motion is lotion.

Conditioning your body the right way can radically reduce stiffness upon standing. You CAN train your body to move without pain. Yes, this will depend on your current condition. If you have sustained serious damage, you may not become completely pain-free, yet there are always improvements you can achieve when you know the right things to do and do them the right way. What do you have to lose by trying?

I remember a patient, Vicky, who had a long, very complicated history. She'd been in several car accidents, resulting in multiple injuries. Vicky had a hip replacement in her early 40s due to injury. She was in constant pain and had very limited function and quality of life. Due to pain, she did less and less until the point when she mostly spent her days in bed. I'll never forget the day she came into the clinic, excited to tell me she'd started doing some simple movements and her pain had lessened by over 30 percent! She was so excited over this result, she practically glowed. Mind you, I'd been attempting to get her to move for many months without success. This change came about when she changed her mindset. She decided she needed to do something and then did it. Mindset matters.

If you haven't completed the Movement Performance Assessment (MPA), I highly recommend it. You'll have a better understanding of your current condition and then the movement education class will introduce you to movement that restores function without pain when you apply all appropriate modifications. You'll learn to load and unload for real-life function. Now, it's up to you …

Strategy #2: FOOD

The next valuable strategy is to ensure the food you put in your mouth is mostly positive with very little negative. I'm not talking about moderation. I believe that word is from the pit of hell as it's caused a lot of damage in daily life decisions. Let me explain.

When you go to mainstream websites, such as the Academy for Nutrition and Dietetics (AND) site, you'll see LOTS of ambiguous words used in lieu of the term moderation. You'll see eat less of this or more of that. You'll see advice to increase this or decrease that. ALL of these statements are very unclear and leave the viewer confused as to the answer they're seeking. You need guidance that provides clarity, not confusion. The REAL question is "how much, how often?" Let's make this clear!

Let me provide clarity that is based on not only the largest study ever done on diet and health; but also on the success of many health care professionals seeing their patients and clients eliminate the need for medications, restore health, and alleviate chronic pain. Yes, I've seen this over and over and over again for nearly 15 years of consulting with people for their health and observing experts in the field who've been successful for 30, 40, even 50 years.

Here's the shorthand version:

A low-fat, whole-food, plant-based diet is key to achieving a long, vibrant, healthy lifespan. I know the confusion out there due to so many conflicting opinions and best-selling books has caused a lot of havoc and angry debates among the general population. I want to state right now, I'm basing this information on seeing people literally reverse conditions like diabetes and CVD and eliminate the need for meds.

I've seen people age really stinkin' well by eating this way. They have great blood work without meds, and their doctors tell them to keep doing what they're doing. I've seen this work, up close and personal, for years and years. I've worked with many people over 100 years of age and seen what was in their kitchen while doing a homecare visit. Those with high quality lives ate a healthy plant-based diet. They weren't necessarily vegan but they ate lots of fruits and veggies, drank water, and kept active movement in their lives.

Being vegan is optional as the data (and real-life examples) show minimizing animal food intake to 10 percent or less is seen to radically lower risk for all those things no one wants, like Type 2 diabetes, cardiovascular disease, and so on. This equates to no more than two to three times a week, not two to three times a day. No ambiguity here. Specifics are key to success.

If you've been eating an animal-based diet for a long time and have been diagnosed with chronic degenerative conditions, you may see speedier improvements by completely eliminating animal foods. Conditions that have led to prescription meds will often respond quicker when your food intake is 100 percent plant-based.

There are some caveats important for you to remember from earlier chapters. Oils injure the cells that line your blood vessels. Injury to those cells leads to lots of things you don't want to happen, such as high blood pressure, heart attacks, and strokes. If you've read the other chapters, you've read the details.

And no, you don't need to graze on your back lawn. Real food is the norm when eating this way. Real food, not something you need to go to a specialty store to get that you've never had before.

If you want to age well and live free of disease for lifelong wellbeing, that power is in your hands and your knife and fork.

I provided four-course meals at my Nourish Away Pain classes taught at the local community college for years. Everyone raved about the food and often ate second helpings, sometimes thirds. They made the recipes at home and loved how much their families enjoyed them as well. The best part? They would share with me how their pain decreased, their A1C improved, and their migraines stopped. I could go on and on but that would be testimonials. Thankfully, the data support this way of eating over and over again.

The Resources section provides some of the recipes people loved in those classes. Simple, real food that is quick and easy to cook. What's not to love?!

I love this quote from *Time Magazine*, October 2003, written by David Bjerklie:

> *"The news is not that fruits and vegetables are good for you, it's that they are so good for you they could save your life."*

Strategy #3: WATER

The third valuable strategy is to ensure you're well hydrated. This means drinking water. Even though you may detest the "taste" of water, it's life-giving.

Dehydration of just 2 percent fluid loss can cause fatigue, decreased blood flow to muscles, reduced endurance, and less than optimal results from exercise. Serious dehydration leads to organ failure, heat stroke, and seizures.

I've heard many people say they choose to limit their water intake because it means they'll need to use the bathroom more often. My response is always the same. *"This is how it works. Water in. Water out."* If you have unwanted leakage issues, please read chapter 5.

Sadly, in nursing home settings, because residents need assistance for bathroom trips and facilities can be short-staffed, many opt to not drink water so they don't need to use their call bell and then wait for what seems like forever for help to arrive. Nobody wants to experience the need to be "cleaned up" because they couldn't wait that long.

On a side note, this is not a criticism of staff or facilities. I could go into many details of why this issue exists, but I don't want to digress from the topic at hand. Hopefully, this will motivate you to actively work to prevent going to a nursing home.

Back to drinking water. Every cell in your body needs water.

If you're drinking coffee or tea in the morning, again at lunch, more in the afternoon (as a pick-me-up), and a cocktail or wine with dinner, you're dehydrating your body 24/7.

Caffeine and alcohol are diuretics. They inhibit your anti-diuretic hormone (ADH), literally tricking your body into thinking it has more water than it needs and you urinate frequently. You may even notice an incontinence issue, like urgency, occurring.

It's a serious problem if you're not replacing the lost water yet continue to have another coffee, cola, or wine. You're simply tricking your body again and losing more water, again!

Statistically, 75 percent of Americans don't drink enough water, and this fact may apply to half the world's population! There are so many reasons your body needs water that this could easily be an entire chapter on just this one topic.

We've known this for 75 years. Our bodies are around 60 percent water!

Sweating, breathing, living ... you lose water all the time; therefore, it needs to be replaced daily:

- Blood plasma is 90 percent water and makes up half your total blood volume
- Your muscles are 78 percent water
- Your lungs are 83 percent water
- Your brain is 73 percent water
- Your bones are 31 percent water

If you want to strengthen your muscles, they need water as much as they need calories, carbs, and resistance training.

Water transports oxygen to your cells, removes waste, and protects your joints and organs. Your body even needs water to regulate body temperature!

Believe it or not, not drinking enough water can even sabotage your weight management goals. The more hydrated you are, the more efficiently your body works at burning body fat.

How do you know if you're not drinking enough water? The easiest way to know is if you're thirsty. I know this may sound ridiculously simple, but the fact is if you're thirsty, you're dehydrated, and your body needed water long before the thirst occurred.

If you don't drink water and you're not feeling thirsty, please know it's reported that in one-third of Americans, the thirst mechanism is so weak it's often mistaken for hunger! You may be adding pounds to the scale by eating more food simply because you need water!

You'll also know you're not drinking enough water if there's a strong odor to your urine, along with a dark yellow or amber color. Urine that shows you're getting an adequate amount of water is colorless or very pale in color, clear, and almost odorless.

There are differing opinions on how to determine how much water you actually need for health. A good estimate is to divide your body weight (in pounds) in half and that number is the number of ounces you need to drink. For example: if you weigh 180 pounds you need 90 ounces of water daily.

I need to add a word of caution if you have decreased kidney function. If your kidneys are unable to eliminate excess water, you can develop an electrolyte imbalance, which can lead to a condition called hyponatremia. Please check with your doctor before taking this step if you have any kidney issues.

In general, drinking too much water is very rare in otherwise healthy adults. Simply stick to half your body weight in pounds to ounces consumed.

If you're not used to drinking water, a simple and easy way to ensure you're getting the amount of water your body requires daily is to divide the amount you need by 16 (waking hours) and drink that amount every 30 minutes. For example, if you require 70 ounces of water (based on a 140-pound body weight) you would drink around 4.5 ounces of water every 30 minutes. Or, to make it even easier, drink just 3 ounces of water every 20 minutes. That is literally just a couple of swallows of water three times an hour. It is quite possible to drink what your body needs without feeling like you're floating away!

Please don't chug a quart of water at the end of the day because you forgot to hydrate during the day. Set your phone to remind you. Get an app that "rewards" you by filling up a body outline as you drink throughout the day.

Louise, a dear friend of mine in her 80s, never drank water. She told me she wasn't thirsty. I was concerned for her because she would spend hours in the sun working on her raspberry patch. She eventually appeased me by drinking more water. Guess what? She was amazed at how she suddenly became thirsty during the day. She literally "reset" her thirst mechanism.

Strategy #4: BELIEF

The last strategy I'll emphasize is your belief system. Yes, your belief system. If you read chapter 1, you now realize the impact your belief system has on your decisions and actions. If we were in the same room right now, I would love to ask you what you believe about the strategies presented in this chapter. Do you believe movement would be helpful to you or do you believe it may make things worse or it's not worth trying?

How about the strategy to nourish your body well? Are you in the high-protein/low-carb camp and your mindset is fixed that's the only way to health? Maybe you "tried" changing your diet, but it didn't seem to help, or it was too much of a learning curve to accomplish, or your family members made it too challenging.

What was your thought reaction to improving your water intake? Did you reject it immediately because of some article you read that told you drinking water was hype? Or do you struggle with unwanted leakage and the last thing you want is more of that?!

If you don't believe you can (or should) do anything about your issues because there are too many obstacles, you're right.

If you believe you can alter your future for the better, you're right. Remember Vicky? Mindset matters.

Which belief do you hold?

The best part? You can CHANGE your belief. This is why I have video resources. You must SEE it to believe it. Now that I think about it, this strategy maybe needs to be first in this chapter …

CHAPTER 12

Methods and Techniques That Work when More Help Is Needed

MYTH: You've tried everything.

In my last book, *Pain Culprits!*, I provided a chapter on the manual techniques and self-care methods I've seen work really well to help people get free from pain and restore life. A reviewer commented that I only shared what could be done with professionals and did not fulfill the subtitle of the book, which is *Surprising Truths Behind Pain, How to Uncover the Cause, and What to do About It.*

It seems that person didn't read the other chapters that provide common causes of many pain issues, why treatment often fails, how everything's connected, and what works.

I even provide a free website with more resources, how to find someone skilled to see you as a whole body, downloads and video instructions to assess yourself to find the culprits causing the pain, AND how to begin training to resolve the issue. One person complained, stating in a review, it made her dizzy to read there was someplace else to go for more information. Really. She complained about getting FREE additional resources and FREE video movement education. You can't make this stuff up!

I share this not to complain about reviews, but to ensure you're aware if this is the only chapter you choose to read, you're missing the whole point of the book, which is to teach you what you need to know and what you need to do. This chapter is provided as a benefit and convenience if you don't have my first book.

This information will be helpful if your needs go beyond what you can do independently, or in case you're confused or stuck and need some expert education or treatment. This way you'll also know what specialty to seek out or what questions to ask of the professionals you're already seeing.

WARNING!

There's no professional or expert clinician who can create or restore full function in your body. I repeat, no person can provide you with good health, pain-free movement, and joyful aging. That can't be done by someone's hands or needles, or meds, or … That work is required from the inside out.

The success you're seeking is not achieved by people working on you from the outside in. They may be helpful in your journey, but they can't bring you to your end goal. I hope this makes sense.

Remember Sue from chapter 4 and her lack of progress because she was counting on everyone else to "fix" her? There's no magic pill, potion, or expert …

Now onto the topic at hand. Let's break this down into two parts.

Part 1 provides methods and knowledge you can learn and apply independently as good self-care for results that work, with results you can experience immediately. This is what "floats my boat" most in my work. I LOVE teaching people how to fix themselves, and these methods work!

Part 2 provides techniques skilled clinicians and experts can provide that are effective with no potential harm and only potential benefit. Experts with experience, training, and knowledge that works without meds and surgery. I know. I use them in my practice.

Part 1: Independent Self-Care Methods

I believe in teaching a person how to fish, which means they aren't dependent on me and my manual skills to address their issues every time they occur. Educating people about how to "fix themselves" is what gets me pumped every day as I train private consults, teach live classes, host events, create online content, and write articles and books.

There are four primary strategies I've seen work in real life to set people free from chronic conditions and pain. You may not need to learn all of them to see relief, but I want to be sure you know about them.

The first and most important thing is what you put in your mouth and whether you are well hydrated. Please read chapter 9 for more on that topic.

The other three methods or concepts, whatever you want to call them, can be amazingly effective at restoring your body to a pain-free state. AND you can learn in the comfort of your own home!

Move Without Pain™

What I'm about to share with you is what has provided more "job" satisfaction than I could ever have imagined over the last 15 years. I began training in Applied Functional Science™ through the Gray Institute after being introduced to the principles behind it in a local clinic where I worked part-time. I was ecstatic as this knowledge about movement was what I'd been searching for my entire career. I saw it as the "Holy Grail" if you will of exercise and movement rehabilitation.

Education in human movement, which I've sought to learn thoroughly since 2009, addresses three critical truths you must know in order to move without pain as you age.

They are:

- Understanding everything is connected to everything else. You're not a knee or a shoulder. You're a whole person.

- Exercise must be done in all three planes of movement to restore or maintain healthy function, strength, and balance. Most exercises are taught in only one.
- All movement training must be authentic. Performing movements your body isn't designed to do and attempting to isolate muscles or body parts repetitively will not breed success long-term and can potentially cause dysfunction and injury.

I covered this more in depth in chapter 10 in case you skipped that chapter.

Because the Gray Institute (GI) teaches health care and movement professionals, I became passionate about teaching these principles and movement truths to the public. I'm not an instructor for the GI, and my program is not one of their trainings. I saw how much this knowledge could change lives when I taught a class based on the principles at the local community college. This is what spurred me to create the Move Without Pain (MWP) Private Club.

This isn't self-promotion to get you to buy something. There is free membership offered in the club AND I have many, many movement education videos on my YouTube channel that cost you nothing but your time to view them. I really want people to know this stuff!

Please check out the Movement Performance Assessment to see how your body is functioning in all three planes of motion. You just may find the culprit causing your pain is not where your pain is happening. Don't you think it's important to know the cause so you can finally resolve any existing pain in your body? If you've tried "everything" but this, you really must check it out.

The success I've seen with people learning and training in authentic three-plane motion has been nothing short of exceptional. I must share an email I received just today from someone in the Have Lifelong Wellbeing Academy so you can see the impact doing the right things the right way can have.

"Just yesterday, we visited with our granddaughter, who has just started walking on her own (mostly, lol) and I was able to get down on the floor with her to play "up and

down" [a peek-a-boo variant], walk with her down the porch steps and pick her up to watch the butterflies ("byes") with more "ups & downs." Ah, the wonderful games one plays with a beginning toddler. All that and more without the pain I used to endure and all because of you!!!"

This is why I do what I do.

Total Motion Release® (TMR)

Total Motion Release is a concept that began in 2002 with Tom Dalonzo-Baker, a highly skilled PT, who found moving and exercising a body part opposite the painful part could be very effective in relieving pain and restoring motion. Often dramatic improvements are seen the first time it's performed.

I first trained in this method years ago and used it successfully in the clinic setting, with virtual consults in countries all over the world, and in classes at the local college.

I remember a woman I saw in the clinic while her therapist was on vacation. Brenda had had left shoulder surgery several weeks prior. She also had a 9-inch jagged scar down the back of her left arm from an old gunshot wound. Talk about a traumatized limb!

Brenda could only lift her left arm a few inches with moderate to severe pain. After performing one set of TMR exercises with her right arm, she was able to lift her left arm much higher with less pain. A second set performed again with her right arm enabled her to lift her left arm nearly straight up to the ceiling with almost no pain.

Her jaw practically hit the floor in disbelief! Even I was amazed! I LOVE this stuff!

More information about TMR is in Resources.

The MELT Method®

MELT was created by Sue Hitzmann, a manual and connective tissue specialist. Sue is also an exercise physiologist, a founding member of the Fascia Research Society, and author of two New York Times-bestselling books *The MELT Method* and *MELT Performance.* Using specialized techniques, a soft body roller, and four small balls of different sizes and densities, MELT is a self-care method that treats and restores your fascial system in a very effective manner. The first clinical study regarding the effect of the MELT Method® on back pain showed significantly decreased pain and a significant increase in flexibility.[1]

I've seen students start crying in local college classes because they could lie on the floor with no pain for the first time in years after performing only ten minutes of MELT techniques. It's even helped me. Before I trained in MELT, I had right shoulder pain from lifting my heavy clinician bag to and from the passenger seat of my car many times a day for ten years while working in homecare.

I could not even push open a door with that arm without intense pain. Nothing I did worked to resolve the problem until I took the level-two MELT instructor training course in Manhattan. My shoulder was pain-free within just three days of training. I couldn't wait to return to work and teach this to others!

You can learn this method via their YouTube channel, their MELT on Demand App, or through one of their many highly trained instructors. I teach a monthly MELT class online as well. Check out the Resources for more information.

Suffice it to say, we must train and treat our bodies in a way that challenges us, nourishes us, strengthens us, and heals us. This requires a multi-prong approach to ensure effective self-care. I highly recommend three-plane training in weight-bearing and effective fascial system self-care. I plan to live to *at least* 112 and be really stinkin' happy about it! Do you want to join me?

Are you willing to learn and do what it takes to age well? Will you be dancing into your 90s and beyond? It doesn't take three hours/day in the gym to do this. You simply need to know the right things to do and then do them.

Part 2: Manual Techniques and Expert Clinicians

I want to begin with a basic reminder. There's no person on the planet who can bring your body to optimal physical function. The only person who can achieve a strong, mobile, pain-free body is you. By that, I mean you must do the work to get you there.

There are no magic shortcuts! Another person cannot make your muscles stronger or make them perform correctly. They can help if there is a problem from an injury or imbalance, but they can't, I repeat, they can't, do the work for you that your body needs to do to fully restore function. Experts can work on you externally to help alleviate pain and improve joint alignment, but the real work to bring you long term success must be done by you. I hope this makes sense.

Biomechanical function, which is how your muscles and joints are working, can be impaired from injuries or accidents. If you're experiencing pain (other than inflammation or nerve injury), it can be due to abnormal muscle tension that creates impaired joint alignment during movement. This can lead to abnormal wear and tear and damage to structures over time.

Abnormal muscle tension impacting joint motion can occur for years because your body is designed to compensate and use other joints and motions to provide what is needed for day-to-day living. This compensation leads to pain over time as structures become irritated, overworked, and ultimately injured.

Muscle Energy Technique (MET)

One of my very favorite and most effective techniques I've used to restore healthy joint alignment is the Muscle Energy Technique. A colleague[2] who has taught this technique for decades is fond of saying, "bone is the slave of muscle." This means restoring healthy muscle function positively impacts joint movement and alleviates pain.

MET was first developed and applied by Fred Mitchell Sr., DO, in 1948. A widely performed and very gentle osteopathic technique, MET is quite effective in improving range of motion restrictions of the neck,[3,4] rib cage,[5] back,[6] pelvis,[7] and extremities.[8,9] It's performed by precise positioning followed by gently contracting specific muscles to improve joint alignment and function.

Mulligan's Mobilizations with Movement (MWMs)

Another of my favorite techniques is Mobilizations with Movement, which was developed in 1983 by Brian Mulligan, PT. I've seen this technique achieve what was often perceived as a miracle by patients in the clinic. MWMs use passive mobilization with active movement. This means the clinician places precise pressure on a joint as the patient actively moves the body part.

This technique often restores pain-free motion in just one to a few treatments. MWMs can be used for any painful orthopedic condition where a limited range of motion is a problem. It's well known to be useful for cervicogenic headaches,[10] neck and back pain,[11] shoulder pain or impingement,[12] hip and knee pain,[13] ankle sprains,[14,15] and tennis or golfer's elbow.[16]

There's a study showing this technique provided benefits to local and widespread pain, physical function (walking), knee flexion and extension muscle strength and knee flexion range of motion (ROM) for at least two days in patients with knee OA.[17] I know two days doesn't seem like much, but the study was looking at this particular technique to see if it would impact knee OA. There was no other intervention provided. No food intake changes or anything else.

Strain and Counterstrain (SCS)

Strain and Counterstrain, also called Positional Release by some, was developed by Lawrence Jones, DO, in 1964 after discovering a muscle positioned in a maximally shortened position for 90 seconds (120 seconds for neurological issues) alleviated pain. A muscle can actively contract (sometimes for years) and promote pain, but passively shortening it in a specific way will allow it to relax.

Passive positioning means you need someone to move your limb without using any muscles to assist the movement. SCS is effective in alleviating pain anywhere there are muscles.[18–20] I love this technique for sciatic pain caused by a piriformis (deep butt muscle) spasm once any sacral issue has been resolved with MET.

There's also an advanced use of this technique developed by Sharon Weiselfish-Giammatteo, PT, that impacts circulatory function, vocal cord function, and much more. I've used both SCS and advanced SCS to improve many issues successfully. Things like vertigo, chronic pain anywhere in the body, pelvic floor pain, and so on.

Trigger Point Therapy (TPT)

Trigger Point Therapy has been studied and performed to address pain for over half a century. It was successfully performed (via injection into trigger points) on President John F. Kennedy to alleviate low back and leg pain by Janet Travell, MD, his personal physician (before and during his White House reign).

A trigger point is a micro-spasm in a muscle and painful to touch. Each trigger point has a specific pain pattern, mapped out by pioneers Dr. Janet Travell and Dr. David Simons, who studied this issue extensively for years and authored manuals well known by manual practitioners.[21]

Muscles have something called spindles, which have two main jobs. One is to set the length and tension of your muscles. The other is to protect muscles from over-stretching and damaging joints. It's this protective mechanism that's responsible for the pain as it can be stuck on and limit motion.

TPT can significantly relieve both acute and chronic pain. When this tiny portion of the muscle gets stuck contracted, the pain created is often in an area far from the trigger point.[22]

The technique should not hurt when done properly. A gentle 90-second, pain-free technique followed by neuromuscular stretching, taught by Dr. Jonathon Kuttner, can be very effective. His book *You Pain Free* is highly recommended for those affected by chronic pain. Injections, dry needling, and acupuncture are also used in trigger point therapy, but self-treatment can be extremely successful resolving pain.[23–26]

Myofascial Release (MFR)

Myofascial Release has been extensively used by massage therapists and bodyworkers, yet there are many physical and occupational therapists trained in MFR as well. Fascia is a type of connective tissue that envelops, surrounds, and protects muscles, vessels, nerves, organs, bones, and so on. It's a continuous fluid structure from head to toe without interruption right down to the cellular level.

Anatomy books state we have around 600 muscles depending on which book you read. I like to explain the importance of fascia this way. *"You don't have hundreds of muscles. You have one muscle separated by hundreds of compartments of fascia."* Treating the fascial system in one area has both a local effect where you're working and a global effect on the entire system.

MFR specifically targets restrictions that occur due to trauma, surgery, scars, and inflammatory responses. These restrictions can produce tensile pressures on pain sensitive structures leading to pain, impaired range of motion, and dysfunction. Treatment applies gentle sustained pressure into (or away from) the myofascial restrictions. Gentle, slow pressure is essential to allow the fascia to elongate and "release."

This technique is never painful if performed by a well trained clinician. Fascia can be treated effectively when surgical scars limit range of motion and create pain.[27] It can also be used for joint, muscle, back[28] and neck pain, headaches, scoliosis,[29] pelvic floor pain, fibromyalgia,[30] and more.[31,32] Fascial restrictions and pain can also be addressed using hands-off self-care, called the MELT Method® presented earlier in this chapter.

McKenzie Method

The McKenzie Method is more a hands-off patient education in movement with only an occasional potential need for the therapist's manual input. This method is defined as a mechanical diagnosis and therapy (MTD) method that uses a classification system[33] to treat back and neck pain.[34–37] There is also treatment for shoulder and knee pain. It was developed in 1981 by

Robin McKenzie, a PT from New Zealand, and is based on the premise of three mechanical syndromes: postural, dysfunction, and derangement.

The power of this method to resolve pain from bulging or herniated discs is phenomenal. I've seen this treatment, when appropriate, eliminate severe pain caused by disc issues in a single session, especially if the problem is classified as a derangement. The patient is required to be very compliant, performing specific motions and restricting certain activities for their exact syndrome to resolve the issue permanently. Once resolved, ongoing attention to not repeat what caused the issue is also taught.

I worked with a young man in his 30s who could barely walk due to severe pain from a herniated disc injury sustained at work while lifting a heavy barrel. Sam was adamantly against surgery, recommended by his orthopedist, and determined to return to work without restrictions. In just three weeks, he was completely free of pain and back to work lifting heavy without restrictions. It was this method and his consistent compliance that accomplished this feat despite the fact experts believed surgery was necessary.

This is not the only case I can relay to you, but I think you get the idea. Surgery is not always the only solution to a problem. Knowing other options is important to make an informed decision.

Hopefully, you've learned a great deal about what works effectively for pain and aging without decline sans all the risks and side effects of drugs and surgery.

Lastly, a conclusion to encourage you …

Conclusion

You've done the first part. You read the book.
Now, are you open to doing the work?

Are you willing to:

- Believe you can age with joy?
  - Reject the myths and misconceptions promoted about aging?
  - Ask yourself those three all-important questions in chapter 1?
- Make changes to your diet?
  - Learn new recipes?
  - Stand out at family gatherings by bringing a dish that nourishes your endothelial cells (like BBQ Beans and Rice) and forgo the four-cheese mac and cheese dish?
- Condition and train your body in three-plane authentic motion?
  - Perform the MPA?
  - Get up consistently throughout your day and do ten simple back bends (to open front hips) and ten chair squats (to bring blood flow to Max)?
- Learn how to do what's needed to move without pain and age without decline?
  - Go to Resources at the *Aging Culprits!* website?
  - Consult with an expert if needed to breed success?

Pretty much everyone CAN do this. The fact is, not everyone WILL do this.

Let me conclude this book with an email I received a while ago from Cheri (by permission):

"Hi, I have a very long history and have been struggling so much for the past four years. When I start telling someone my history, it sounds like a joke. Like there is no way that all of this could have and still be happening to one person.

"Anyway, I have to tell you that in doing the three-day challenge and the work that I have done since joining the academy, I feel amazing. I am not where I want to be but, I feel that there may be hope now. Thank you for all that you do."

Here's a follow up email sent less than a month later:

"Eileen, I just want you to know how very happy I am with the program … I have noticed quite a difference in everything on my body. My knee pain is also gone.

"You have definitely put your heart and soul into it and I am so glad that I finally joined. I just wanted to let you know."

Cheri

About the Author

Eileen Kopsaftis, BS, PT, FAFS, CMI, NE has been helping people resolve pain and age well since 1994 in settings such as nursing homes, long-term rehab, homecare, hospitals, and orthopedic outpatient. She has spent thirty years researching and seeking truths related to pain and aging. Eileen's approach has empowered hundreds of people to literally reverse many of the common "symptoms" of aging such as joint pain, poor balance, stooped posture, muscle loss, and the need for disposable underwear. Her approach is based on the mostly unknown truths of human movement, powerful self-care methods, and science-based nutrition education combined.

Eileen's passion is to teach people how to radically reduce the risk of ending up in a nursing home. This led to the creation of the Have Lifelong Wellbeing Academy to equip people to successfully age without pain and decline. She truly believes we all can have lifelong well-being.

www.agingculprits.com

Resources

This is my favorite part of the book as I get to give you MORE.

More information. More knowledge.

Not just *what* to do, but *how* to do it successfully. Woo Hoo!

Simply go to AgingCulprits.com and you'll find resources mentioned in each chapter with clickable links and downloads.

There's even email support if you have any trouble finding anything because your success is important to me:

Support@HaveLifelongWellbeing.com

References

Chapter 1

1. Robertson, Claire E., Nicolas Pröllochs, Kaoru Schwarzenegger, Philip Pärnamets, Jay J. Van Bavel, and Stefan Feuerriegel. 2023. "Negativity Drives Online News Consumption." *Nature Human Behaviour* 7 (5): 812–22. https://doi.org/10.1038/s41562-023-01538-4.
2. Ewen, Heidi H., Katherina Nikzad-Terhune, and Kara B. Dassel. 2020. "Exploring Beliefs About Aging and Faith: Development of the Judeo-Christian Religious Beliefs and Aging Scale." *Behavioral Sciences* 10 (9): 139. https://doi.org/10.3390/bs10090139.
3. Levy, Becca R., Martin D. Slade, and Stanislav V. Kasl. 2002. "Longitudinal Benefit of Positive Self-Perceptions of Aging on Functional Health." *Journals of Gerontology Series B* 57 (5): 409–17. https://doi.org/10.1093/geronb/57.5.p409.
4. Levy, Becca R., Alan B. Zonderman, Martin D. Slade, and Luigi Ferrucci. 2009. "Age Stereotypes Held Earlier in Life Predict Cardiovascular Events in Later Life." *Psychological Science* 20 (3): 296–98. https://doi.org/10.1111/j.1467-9280.2009.02298.x.

Chapter 2

1. WebMD Editorial Contributor. 2023. "Common Medications for Older Adults." WebMD. April 7, 2023. https://www.webmd.com/healthy-aging/common-medications-for-older-adults.
2. Sun, WeiPing, HaiBin Zhang, JinCheng Guo, XueKun Zhang, LiXin Zhang, ChunLei Li, and Ling Zhang. 2016. "Comparison of the Efficacy and Safety of Different ACE Inhibitors in Patients With Chronic Heart Failure." *Medicine* 95 (6): e2554. https://doi.org/10.1097/md.0000000000002554. PMID: 26871774; PMCID: PMC4753869.
3. Barnard, R J. 1991. "Effects of Life-style Modification on Serum Lipids." *Archives of Internal Medicine* 151 (7): 1389. https://doi.org/10.1001/archinte.1991.00400070141019.
4. Saunders, T. 1983. "Dietary fat and platelet function." *Clinical Science* 65: 343. https://pdfs.semanticscholar.org/cbe1/3a1767de7c9064f5be0e66e8e636fb4d5a59.pdf.
5. Parke-Davis. n.d. "Product Information. Lipitor (atorvastatin)." Morris Plains, NJ: Parke-Davis.
6. Cerner Multum, Inc. "Australian Product Information."

7. Arora, Rohit, Max Liebo, and Frank Maldonado. 2006. "Statin-Induced Myopathy: The Two Faces of Janus." *Journal of Cardiovascular Pharmacology and Therapeutics* 11 (2): 105–12. https://doi.org/10.1177/1074248406288758.

8. Plosker, Greg L., and Donna McTavish. 1995. "Simvastatin: A Reappraisal of its Pharmacology and Therapeutic Efficacy in Hypercholesterolaemia." *Drugs* 50 (2): 334–63. https://doi.org/10.2165/00003495-199550020-00009.

9. Bilheimer, David W. 1990. "Long-Term Clinical Tolerance of Lovastatin and Simvastatin." *Cardiology* 77 (4): 58–65. https://doi.org/10.1159/000174684.

10. Sanson, Gillian. 2003. *The Myth of Osteoporosis. What Every Woman Should Know about Creating Bone Health.* Ann Arbor MI: MCD Publications, 37.

11. Cumming, R.G., and R.J. Klineberg. 1994. "Case-Control Study of Risk Factors for Hip Fractures in the Elderly." *American Journal of Epidemiology* 139 (5): 493–503. https://doi.org/10.1093/oxfordjournals.aje.a117032.

12. Marshall, D., O. Johnell, and H. Wedel. 1996. "Meta-analysis of How Well Measures of Bone Mineral Density Predict Occurrence of Osteoporotic Fractures." *Maturitas* 25 (2): 157–58. https://doi.org/10.1016/0378-5122(96)81789-0.

13. Cummings, S. R., D. M. Black, D. E. Thompson, W. B. Applegate, E. Barrett-Connor, T. A. Musliner, L. Palermo, et al. 1998. "Effect of Alendronate on Risk of Fracture in Women With Low Bone Density but Without Vertebral Fractures: Results From the Fracture Intervention Trial." *JAMA* 280 (24): 2077. https://doi.org/10.1001/jama.280.24.2077.

14. Mashiba, Tasuku, Toru Hirano, Charles H. Turner, Mark R. Forwood, C. Conrad Johnston, and David B. Burr. 2000. "Suppressed Bone Turnover by Bisphosphonates Increases Microdamage Accumulation and Reduces Some Biomechanical Properties in Dog Rib." *Journal of Bone and Mineral Research* 15 (4): 613–20. https://doi.org/10.1359/jbmr.2000.15.4.613.

15. Neviaser, Andrew S., Joseph M. Lane, Brett A. Lenart, Folorunsho Edobor-Osula, and Dean G. Lorich. 2008. "Low-Energy Femoral Shaft Fractures Associated With Alendronate Use." *Journal of Orthopaedic Trauma* 22 (5): 346–50. https://doi.org/10.1097/bot.0b013e318172841c.

16. Schilcher, Jörg, Veronika Koeppen, Per Aspenberg, and Karl Michaëlsson. 2015. "Risk of Atypical Femoral Fracture During and After Bisphosphonate Use." *Acta Orthopaedica* 86 (1): 100–107. https://doi.org/10.3109/17453674.2015.1004149. PMID: 25582459; PMCID: PMC4366670.

17. Sedghizadeh, Parish P., Kyle Stanley, Matthew Caligiuri, Shawn Hofkes, Brad Lowry, and Charles F. Shuler. 2009. "Oral Bisphosphonate Use and the Prevalence of Osteonecrosis of the Jaw: An Institutional Inquiry." *Journal of the American Dental Association* 140 (1): 61–66. https://doi.org/10.14219/jada.archive.2009.0019.

18. Miller, Paul D., Gary Hattersley, Bente Juel Riis, Gregory C. Williams, Edith Lau, Luis Augusto Russo, Peter Alexandersen, et al. 2016. "Effect of Abaloparatide vs Placebo on New Vertebral Fractures in Postmenopausal Women with Osteoporosis." *JAMA* 316 (7): 722–33. https://doi.org/10.1001/jama.2016.11136.

19. FDA. "FORTEO® teriparatide (rDNA origin) injection 750 mcg/3 mL." www.accessdata.fda.gov/drugsatfda_docs/label/2008/021318s015lbl.pdf.

20. Cosman, Felicia, Daria B. Crittenden, Jonathan D. Adachi, Neil Binkley, Edward Czerwinski, Serge Ferrari, Lorenz C. Hofbauer, et al. 2016. "Romosozumab Treatment in Postmenopausal Women With Osteoporosis." *New England Journal of Medicine* 375 (16): 1532–43. https://doi.org/10.1056/nejmoa1607948.

21. Towheed, Tanveer, Lara Maxwell, Maria Judd, Michelle Catton, Marc C Hochberg, and George A Wells. 2006. "Acetaminophen for Osteoarthritis." *Cochrane Library* 2010 (1). https://doi.org/10.1002/14651858.cd004257.pub2.

22. Larson, Anne M., Julie Polson, Robert J. Fontana, Timothy J. Davern, Ezmina Lalani, Linda S. Hynan, Joan S. Reisch, et al. 2005. "Acetaminophen-induced Acute Liver Failure: Results of a United States Multicenter, Prospective Study." *Hepatology* 42 (6): 1364–72. https://doi.org/10.1002/hep.20948.

23. Bjordal, Jan Magnus, Anne Elisabeth Ljunggren, Atle Klovning, and Lars Slørdal. 2004. "Non-steroidal Anti-inflammatory Drugs, Including Cyclo-oxygenase-2 Inhibitors, in Osteoarthritic Knee Pain: Meta-analysis of Randomised Placebo Controlled Trials." *BMJ* 329 (7478): 1317. https://doi.org/10.1136/bmj.38273.626655.63.

24. Singh, G., and G. Triadafilopoulos. 1999. "Epidemiology of NSAID Induced Gastrointestinal Complications." *PubMed* 56 (April): 18–24. https://pubmed.ncbi.nlm.nih.gov/10225536.

25. Liu, Gang, Yu-Peng Yan, Xin-Xin Zheng, Yan-Lu Xu, Jie Lu, Ru-Tai Hui, and Xiao-Hong Huang. 2014. "Meta-Analysis of Nonsteroidal Anti-Inflammatory Drug Use and Risk of Atrial Fibrillation." *American Journal of Cardiology* 114 (10): 1523–29. https://doi.org/10.1016/j.amjcard.2014.08.015.

26. Schnitzer, Thomas J. 2006. "Update on Guidelines for the Treatment of Chronic Musculoskeletal Pain." *Clinical Rheumatology* 25 (S1): 22–29. https://doi.org/10.1007/s10067-006-0203-8.

27. Lilja, M., M. Mandić, W. Apró, M. Melin, K. Olsson, S. Rosenborg, T. Gustafsson, and T. R. Lundberg. 2017. "High Doses of Anti-inflammatory Drugs Compromise Muscle Strength and Hypertrophic Adaptations to Resistance Training in Young Adults." *Acta Physiologica* 222 (2). https://doi.org/10.1111/apha.12948. PMID: 28834248.

28. McAlindon, Timothy E., Michael P. LaValley, William F. Harvey, Lori Lyn Price, Jeffrey B. Driban, Ming Zhang, and Robert J. Ward. 2017. "Effect of Intra-articular Triamcinolone vs Saline on Knee Cartilage Volume and Pain in Patients With Knee Osteoarthritis." *JAMA* 317 (19): 1967. https://doi.org/10.1001/jama.2017.5283.

29. Merck & Co. "Product Information. Cortone Acetate (cortisone)." West Point, PA: Merck & Co, Inc.

30. FDA. 2014. "FDA Drug Safety Communication: FDA Requires Label Changes to Warn of Rare but Serious Neurologic Problems after Epidural Corticosteroid Injections for Pain." www.fda.gov/media/88483/download.

31. Bedson, John, and Peter R. Croft. 2008. "The Discordance Between Clinical and Radiographic Knee Osteoarthritis: A Systematic Search and Summary of the Literature." *BMC Musculoskeletal Disorders* 9 (1). https://doi.org/10.1186/1471-2474-9-116.

32. Singh, Jasvinder A., Shaohua Yu, Lang Chen, and John D. Cleveland. 2019. "Rates of Total Joint Replacement in the United States: Future Projections to 2020–2040 Using the National Inpatient Sample." *Journal of Rheumatology* 46 (9): 1134–40. https://doi.org/10.3899/jrheum.170990. PMID: 30988126.

33. Moseley, J. Bruce, Kimberly O'Malley, Nancy J. Petersen, Terri J. Menke, Baruch A. Brody, David H. Kuykendall, John C. Hollingsworth, Carol M. Ashton, and Nelda P. Wray. 2002. "A Controlled Trial of Arthroscopic Surgery for Osteoarthritis of the Knee." *New England Journal of Medicine* 347 (2): 81–88. https://doi.org/10.1056/nejmoa013259.

34. O'Connor, Denise, Renea V. Johnston, Romina Brignardello-Petersen, Rudolf W. Poolman, Sheila Cyril, Per O. Vandvik, and Rachelle Buchbinder. 2022. "Arthroscopic Surgery for Degenerative Knee Disease (Osteoarthritis Including Degenerative Meniscal Tears)." *Cochrane Library* 2022 (3). https://doi.org/10.1002/14651858.cd014328. PMID: 35238404; PMCID: PMC8892839.

35. Lee, Hahn-Ey, Sung Yong Cho, Sangim Lee, Myong Kim, and Seung-June Oh. 2013. "Short-term Effects of a Systematized Bladder Training Program for Idiopathic Overactive Bladder: A Prospective Study." *International Neurourology Journal* 17 (1): 11. https://doi.org/10.5213/inj.2013.17.1.11.

36. Funada, Satoshi, Takashi Yoshioka, Yan Luo, Akira Sato, Shusuke Akamatsu, and Norio Watanabe. 2023. "Bladder Training for Treating Overactive Bladder in Adults." *Cochrane Library* 2023 (10). https://doi.org/10.1002/14651858.cd013571.pub2. PMID: 37811598; PMCID: PMC10561149.

37. Gandi, Carlo, and Emilio Sacco. 2021. "Pharmacological Management of Urinary Incontinence: Current and Emerging Treatment." *Clinical Pharmacology Advances and Applications* 13 (November): 209–23. https://doi.org/10.2147/cpaa.s289323. PMID: 34858068; PMCID: PMC8630428.

Chapter 3

1. Muniyappa, Ranganath, and James R. Sowers. 2013. "Role of Insulin Resistance in Endothelial Dysfunction." *Reviews in Endocrine and Metabolic Disorders* 14 (1): 5–12. https://doi.org/10.1007/s11154-012-9229-1.

2. Clyne, Alisa Morss. 2021. "Endothelial Response to Glucose: Dysfunction, Metabolism, and Transport." *Biochemical Society Transactions* 49 (1): 313–25. https://doi.org/10.1042/bst20200611. PMID: 33522573; PMCID: PMC7920920.

3. Theofilis, Panagiotis, Marios Sagris, Evangelos Oikonomou, Alexios S. Antonopoulos, Gerasimos Siasos, Costas Tsioufis, and Dimitris Tousoulis. 2021. "Inflammatory Mechanisms Contributing to Endothelial Dysfunction." *Biomedicines* 9 (7): 781. https://doi.org/10.3390/biomedicines9070781. PMID: 34356845; PMCID: PMC8301477.

4. Higashi, Yukihito, Tatsuya Maruhashi, Kensuke Noma, and Yasuki Kihara. 2014. "Oxidative Stress and Endothelial Dysfunction: Clinical Evidence and Therapeutic Implications." *Trends in Cardiovascular Medicine* 24 (4): 165–69. https://doi.org/10.1016/j.tcm.2013.12.001. PMID: 24373981.

5. Su, Jin Bo. 2015. "Vascular Endothelial Dysfunction and Pharmacological Treatment." *World Journal of Cardiology* 7 (11): 719. https://doi.org/10.4330/wjc.v7.i11.719. PMID: 26635921; PMCID: PMC4660468.

6. Blankenhorn, David H. 1990. "The Influence of Diet on the Appearance of New Lesions in Human Coronary Arteries." *JAMA* 263 (12): 1646. https://doi.org/10.1001/jama.1990.03440120068039.

7. Vogel, Robert A., Mary C. Corretti, and Gary D. Plotnick. 2000. "The Postprandial Effect of Components of the Mediterranean Diet on Endothelial Function." *Journal of the American College of Cardiology* 36 (5): 1455–60. https://doi.org/10.1016/s0735-1097(00)00896-2.

8. Felton, C.V., D. Crook, M. J. Davies, and M. F. Oliver. 1994. "Dietary Polyunsaturated Fatty Acids and Composition of Human Aortic Plaques." *The Lancet* 344 (8931): 1195–96. https://doi.org/10.1016/s0140-6736(94)90511-8.

9. Hennig, B., and B A Watkins. 1989. "Linoleic Acid and Linolenic Acid: Effect on Permeability Properties of Cultured Endothelial Cell Monolayers." *American Journal of Clinical Nutrition* 49 (2): 301–5. https://doi.org/10.1093/ajcn/49.2.301.

10. Hooper, Lee, Rachel L. Thompson, Roger A. Harrison, Carolyn D. Summerbell, Andy R. Ness, Helen J. Moore, Helen V. Worthington, et al. 2006. "Risks and Benefits of Omega 3 Fats for Mortality, Cardiovascular Disease, and Cancer: Systematic Review." *BMJ* 332 (7544): 752–60. https://doi.org/10.1136/bmj.38755.366331.2f.

11. Kauppila, L. I. 2009. "Atherosclerosis and Disc Degeneration/Low-Back Pain – A Systematic Review." *European Journal of Vascular and Endovascular Surgery* 37 (6): 661–70. https://doi.org/10.1016/j.ejvs.2009.02.006.

12. Leino-Arjas, Päivi, Leena Kauppila, Leena Kaila-Kangas, Rahman Shiri, Sami Heistaro, and Markku Heliövaara. 2008. "Serum Lipids in Relation to Sciatica Among Finns." *Atherosclerosis* 197 (1): 43–49. https://doi.org/10.1016/j.atherosclerosis.2007.07.035. PMID: 17825307.

13. Leboeuf-Yde, C. 1999. "Smoking and Low Back Pain." *Spine* 24 (14): 1463. https://doi.org/10.1097/00007632-199907150-00012. PMID: 10423792.

14. Goldberg, Mark S., Susan C. Scott, and Nancy E. Mayo. 2000. "A Review of the Association Between Cigarette Smoking and the Development of Nonspecific Back Pain and Related Outcomes." *Spine* 25 (8): 995–1014. https://doi.org/10.1097/00007632-200004150-00016.PMID: 10767814.

15. Hangai, Mika, Koji Kaneoka, Shinya Kuno, Shiro Hinotsu, Masataka Sakane, Naotaka Mamizuka, Shinsuke Sakai, and Naoyuki Ochiai. 2008. "Factors Associated With Lumbar Intervertebral Disc Degeneration in the Elderly." *Spine Journal* 8 (5): 732–40. https://doi.org/10.1016/j.spinee.2007.07.392.

16. García-Gavilán, Jesús Francisco, Alfredo Martínez, Jadwiga Konieczna, Rafael Mico-Perez, Ana García-Arellano, Josep Basora, Laura Barrubés, et al. 2021. "U-Shaped Association Between Dietary Acid Load and Risk of Osteoporotic Fractures in 2 Populations at High Cardiovascular Risk." *Journal of Nutrition* 151 (1): 152–61. https://doi.org/10.1093/jn/nxaa335.

17. Hart, Nicolas H., Robert U. Newton, Jocelyn Tan, Timo Rantalainen, Paola Chivers, Aris Siafarikas, and Sophia Nimphius. 2020. "Biological Basis of Bone Strength: Anatomy, Physiology and Measurement." *Journal of Musculoskeletal & Neuronal Interactions* 20 (3) 2020. https://www.ncbi.nlm.nih.gov/pmc/articles/PMC7493450. PMID: 32877972; PMCID: PMC7493450.

Chapter 4

1. Frontera, Walter R., Virginia A. Hughes, Roger A. Fielding, Maria A. Fiatarone, William J. Evans, and Ronenn Roubenoff. 2000. "Aging of Skeletal Muscle: A 12-yr Longitudinal Study." *Journal of Applied Physiology* 88 (4): 1321–26. https://doi.org/10.1152/jappl.2000.88.4.1321.

2. Saltin, B., G. Blomqvist, J. H. Mitchell, R. L. Johnson Jr., K. Wildenthal, C. B. Chapman. 1968. "Response to Exercise after Bed Rest and after Training." *Circulation* 38 (5 Suppl): VII1–78. https://doi.org/10.7326/0003-4819-71-2-444_1.

3. Melov, Simon, Mark A. Tarnopolsky, Kenneth Beckman, Krysta Felkey, and Alan Hubbard. 2007. "Resistance Exercise Reverses Aging in Human Skeletal Muscle." *PLOS ONE* 2 (5): e465. https://doi.org/10.1371/journal.pone.0000465.PMID: 17520024; PMCID: PMC1866181.

4. Pahor, Marco, Jack M. Guralnik, Walter T. Ambrosius, Steven Blair, Denise E. Bonds, Timothy S. Church, Mark A. Espeland, et al. 2014. "Effect of Structured Physical Activity on Prevention of Major Mobility Disability in Older Adults." *JAMA* 311 (23): 2387. https://doi.org/10.1001/jama.2014.5616.

Chapter 5

1. Gorina, Y., S. Schappert, A. Bercovitz, et al. 2014. "Prevalence of Incontinence among Older Americans." *CDC Vital and Health Statistics* 3 (36). https://www.cdc.gov/nchs/data/series/sr_03/sr03_036.pdf#tab02

2. Tamanini, José Tadeu Nunes, Maria Lúcia Lebrão, Yeda A. O. Duarte, Jair L. F. Santos, and Ruy Laurenti. 2009. "Analysis of the Prevalence of and Factors Associated With Urinary Incontinence Among Elderly People in the Municipality of São Paulo, Brazil: SABE Study (Health, Wellbeing and Aging)." *Cadernos De Saúde Pública* 25 (8): 1756–62. https://doi.org/10.1590/s0102-311x2009000800011.

3. DuBeau, Catherine E., George A. Kuchel, Theodore Johnson II, Mary H. Palmer, and Adrian Wagg. 2009. "Incontinence in the Frail Elderly: Report From the 4th International Consultation on Incontinence." *Neurourology and Urodynamics* 29 (1): 165–78. https://doi.org/10.1002/nau.20842. PMID: 20025027.

4. Sidik, Sherina Mohd. 2010. "The Prevalence of Urinary Incontinence Among the Elderly in a Rural Community in Selangor." *Malaysian Journal of Medical Science* 17 (2): 18–23. https://pubmed.ncbi.nlm.nih.gov/22135533.

5. Leung, Felix W., and John F. Schnelle. 2008. "Urinary and Fecal Incontinence in Nursing Home Residents." *Gastroenterology Clinics of North America* 37 (3): 697–707. https://doi.org/10.1016/j.gtc.2008.06.005. PMID: 18794004; PMCID: PMC2614622.

6. Chong, Julio T., and Vannita Simma-Chiang. 2017. "A Historical Perspective and Evolution of the Treatment of Male Urinary Incontinence." *Neurourology and Urodynamics* 37 (3): 1169–75. https://doi.org/10.1002/nau.23429. PMID: 29053886.

7. Jerez-Roig, Javier, Joanne Booth, Dawn A. Skelton, Maria Giné-Garriga, Sebastien F. M. Chastin, and Suzanne Hagen. 2020. "Is Urinary Incontinence Associated With Sedentary Behaviour in Older Women? Analysis of Data From the National Health and Nutrition Examination Survey." *PLOS ONE* 15 (2): e0227195. https://doi.org/10.1371/journal.pone.0227195.

8. Schumpf, Lea F., Nathan Theill, David A. Scheiner, Daniel Fink, Florian Riese, and Cornelia Betschart. 2017. "Urinary Incontinence and Its Association With Functional Physical and Cognitive Health Among Female Nursing Home Residents in Switzerland." *BMC Geriatrics* 17 (1). https://doi.org/10.1186/s12877-017-0414-7.

Chapter 6

1. Rubenstein, Laurence Z. 2006. "Falls in Older People: Epidemiology, Risk Factors and Strategies for Prevention." *Age And Ageing* 35 (Suppl_2): ii37–41. https://doi.org/10.1093/ageing/afl084.

2. WHO. 2008. *WHO Global Report on Falls Prevention in Older Age*, 1–47. Geneva: World Health Organization. https://www.who.int/publications/i/item/9789241563536.

3. Gell, Nancy M., Robert B. Wallace, Andrea Z. LaCroix, Tracy M. Mroz, and Kushang V. Patel. 2015. "Mobility Device Use in Older Adults and Incidence of Falls and Worry About Falling: Findings From the 2011–2012 National Health and Aging Trends Study." *Journal of the American Geriatrics Society* 63 (5): 853–59. https://doi.org/10.1111/jgs.13393.

4. Thies, Sibylle Brunhilde, Alex Bates, Eleonora Costamagna, Laurence Kenney, Malcolm Granat, Jo Webb, Dave Howard, Rose Baker, and Helen Dawes. 2020. "Are Older People Putting Themselves at Risk When Using Their Walking Frames?" *BMC Geriatrics* 20 (1). https://doi.org/10.1186/s12877-020-1450-2.

5. Hospital for Special Surgery. n.d. "Addressing Falls Prevention Among Older Adults, Part I: Understanding Why Falls Happen." https://www.hss.edu/conditions_addressing-falls-prevention-older-adults-understanding.asp.

6. CDC. 2024. "Older Adult Falls Data." *Older Adult Fall Prevention*. https://www.cdc.gov/falls/data-research/?CDC_AAref_Val=https://www.cdc.gov/falls/data/index.html.

7. Lin, Frank R., and Luigi Ferrucci. 2012. "Hearing Loss and Falls Among Older Adults in the United States." *Archives of Internal Medicine* 172 (4): 369. https://doi.org/10.1001/archinternmed.2011.728. PMID: 22371929; PMCID: PMC3518403.

8. Rogers, Christine. 2021. "Audiologists Should Not Fail With Falls: A Call to Commit to Prevention of Falls in Older Adults." *South African Journal of Communication Disorders* 68 (1). https://doi.org/10.4102/sajcd.v68i1.841. PMID: 34636596; PMCID: PMC8517736.

9. Anand, Vijay, John G. Buckley, Andy Scally, and David B. Elliott. 2003. "Postural Stability in the Elderly During Sensory Perturbations and Dual Tasking: The Influence of Refractive Blur." *Investigative Ophthalmology & Visual Science* 44 (7): 2885. https://doi.org/10.1167/iovs.02-1031.

10. Haines, Michelle. 2015. "3 Nets of Connection." *MELT Method* (blog). January 21, 2015. https://meltmethod.com/blogs/articles/3-nets-connection?zCountry=US.

11. Thomas, Ewan, Giuseppe Battaglia, Antonino Patti, Jessica Brusa, Vincenza Leonardi, Antonio Palma, and Marianna Bellafiore. 2019. "Physical Activity Programs for Balance and Fall Prevention in Elderly." *Medicine* 98 (27): e16218. https://doi.org/10.1097/md.0000000000016218. PMID: 31277132; PMCID: PMC6635278.

Chapter 7

1. Tingen Construction. "The Benefits of a Zero-Entry House." June 2, 2020. https://tingen.com/2020/06/02/the-benefits-of-a-zero-entry-house.

2. Brooks, Rodney. 2018. "Retirement Dream Home Mistakes to Avoid." Money section, *US News and World Report*. July 10, 2018. https://money.usnews.com/money/retirement/baby-boomers/articles/2018-07-10/retirement-dream-home-mistakes-to-avoid.

3. Friedman, Robyn. 2023. "How to Decide Between a One- or Two-Story Home." NewHomeSource.Com. September 26, 2023. https://www.newhomesource.com/learn/two-story-or-one-story-home-plans.

4. Lutz, G. E., R. A. Palmitier, K. N. An, and E. Y. Chao. 1993. "Comparison of Tibiofemoral Joint Forces During Open-kinetic-chain and Closed-kinetic-chain Exercises." *Journal of Bone and Joint Surgery* 75 (5): 732–39. https://doi.org/10.2106/00004623-199305000-00014.

Chapter 8

1. Kang, Na-Yeon, Sang-Cheol Im, and Kyoung Kim. 2021. "Effects of a Combination of Scapular Stabilization and Thoracic Extension Exercises for Office Workers With Forward Head Posture on the Craniovertebral Angle, Respiration, Pain, and Disability: A Randomized-controlled Trial." *Turkish Journal of Physical Medicine and Rehabilitation* 67 (3): 291–99. https://doi.org/10.5606/tftrd.2021.6397. PMID: 34870115; PMCID: PMC8606989.

Chapter 9

1. World Health Organization. 2023. "Dementia." March 15, 2023. https://www.who.int/news-room/fact-sheets/detail/dementia.

2. Dhana, Klodian, Bryan D. James, Puja Agarwal, Neelum T. Aggarwal, Laurel J. Cherian, Sue E. Leurgans, Lisa L. Barnes, David A. Bennett, and Julie A. Schneider. 2021. "MIND Diet, Common Brain Pathologies, and Cognition in Community-Dwelling Older Adults." *Journal of Alzheimer's Disease* 83 (2): 683–92. https://doi.org/10.3233/jad-210107.

3. Morris, Martha Clare, Christy C. Tangney, Yamin Wang, Frank M. Sacks, Lisa L. Barnes, David A. Bennett, and Neelum T. Aggarwal. 2015. "MIND Diet Slows Cognitive Decline With Aging." *Alzheimer's & Dementia* 11 (9): 1015–22. https://doi.org/10.1016/j.jalz.2015.04.011. PMID: 26086182; PMCID: PMC4581900.

4. Gentreau, Mélissa, Virginie Chuy, Catherine Féart, Cécilia Samieri, Karen Ritchie, Michel Raymond, Claire Berticat, and Sylvaine Artero. 2020. "Refined Carbohydrate-rich Diet Is Associated With Long-term Risk of Dementia and Alzheimer's Disease in Apolipoprotein E E4 Allele Carriers." *Alzheimer's & Dementia* 16 (7): 1043–53. https://doi.org/10.1002/alz.12114.

5. Zhang, Huifeng, Darren C. Greenwood, Harvey A. Risch, David Bunce, Laura J. Hardie, and Janet E. Cade. 2021. "Meat Consumption and Risk of Incident Dementia: Cohort Study of 493,888 UK Biobank Participants." *American Journal of Clinical Nutrition* 114 (1): 175–84. https://doi.org/10.1093/ajcn/nqab028. PMID: 33748832; PMCID: PMC8246598.

6. Jia, Jianping, Tan Zhao, Zhaojun Liu, Yumei Liang, Fangyu Li, Yan Li, Wenying Liu, et al. 2023. "Association Between Healthy Lifestyle and Memory Decline in Older Adults: 10 Year, Population Based, Prospective Cohort Study." *BMJ*, January, e072691. https://doi.org/10.1136/bmj-2022-072691. PMID: 36696990; PMCID: PMC9872850.

7. Holstege, Henne, Nina Beker, Tjitske Dijkstra, Karlijn Pieterse, Elizabeth Wemmenhove, Kimja Schouten, Linette Thiessens, et al. 2018. "The 100-plus Study of Cognitively Healthy Centenarians: Rationale, Design and Cohort Description." *European Journal of Epidemiology* 33 (12): 1229–49. https://doi.org/10.1007/s10654-018-0451-3. PMID: 30362018; PMCID: PMC6290855.

8. Martin, S. S., A. W. Aday, Z. I. Almarzooq, C. A. M. Anderson, P. Arora, C. L. Avery, et al. on behalf of the American Heart Association Council on Epidemiology and Prevention Statistics Committee and Stroke Statistics Subcommittee. 2024. "2024 Heart Disease and Stroke Statistics: A Report of US and Global Data from the American Heart Association." *Circulation*. Published online January 24, 2024. https://doi.org.10.1161/CIR.0000000000001209. https://www.heart.org/-/media/PHD-Files-2/Science-News/2/2024-Heart-and-Stroke-Stat-Update/2024-Statistics-At-A-Glance-final_2024.pdf.

9. Blankenhorn, David H. 1990. "The Influence of Diet on the Appearance of New Lesions in Human Coronary Arteries." *JAMA* 263 (12): 1646. https://doi.org/10.1001/jama.1990.03440120068039.

10. Vogel, Robert A., Mary C. Corretti, and Gary D. Plotnick. 2000. "The Postprandial Effect of Components of the Mediterranean Diet on Endothelial Function." *Journal of the American College of Cardiology* 36 (5): 1455–60. https://doi.org/10.1016/s0735-1097(00)00896-2.

11. Felton, C.V., D. Crook, M.J. Davies, and M.F. Oliver. 1994. "Dietary Polyunsaturated Fatty Acids and Composition of Human Aortic Plaques." *The Lancet* 344 (8931): 1195–96. https://doi.org/10.1016/s0140-6736(94)90511-8.

12. Hennig, B., and B. A. Watkins. 1989. "Linoleic Acid and Linolenic Acid: Effect on Permeability Properties of Cultured Endothelial Cell Monolayers." *American Journal of Clinical Nutrition* 49 (2): 301–5. https://doi.org/10.1093/ajcn/49.2.301.

13. Hooper, Lee, Rachel L. Thompson, Roger A. Harrison, Carolyn D. Summerbell, Andy R. Ness, Helen J. Moore, Helen V. Worthington, et al. 2006. "Risks and Benefits of Omega 3 Fats for Mortality, Cardiovascular Disease, and Cancer: Systematic Review." *BMJ* 332 (7544): 752–60. https://doi.org/10.1136/bmj.38755.366331.2f.

14. Wachman, Amnon, and Daniel S. Bernstein. 1968. "Diet and Osteoporosis." *The Lancet* 291 (7549): 958–59. https://doi.org/10.1016/s0140-6736(68)90908-2.

15. Barzel, Uriel S., and Linda K. Massey. 1998. "Excess Dietary Protein Can Adversely Affect Bone." *Journal of Nutrition* 128 (6): 1051–53. https://doi.org/10.1093/jn/128.6.1051.

16. Margen, S., J. Y. Chu, N. A. Kaufmann, and D. H. Calloway. 1974. "Studies in Calcium Metabolism. I. The Calciuretic Effect of Dietary Protein." *American Journal of Clinical Nutrition* 27 (6): 584–89. https://doi.org/10.1093/ajcn/27.6.584.

17. Kerstetter, Jane E., and Lindsay H. Allen. 1990. "Dietary Protein Increases Urinary Calcium," *Journal of Nutrition* 120 (1): 134–6, https://doi.org/10.1093/jn/120.1.134, https://www.sciencedirect.com/science/article/pii/S0022316622174171.

18. Carnauba, Renata, Ana Baptistella, Valéria Paschoal, and Gilberti Hübscher. 2017. "Diet-Induced Low-Grade Metabolic Acidosis and Clinical Outcomes: A Review." *Nutrients* 9 (6): 538. https://doi.org/10.3390/nu9060538. PMID: 28587067; PMCID: PMC5490517.

19. Paterson, C. R. 1978. "Calcium Requirements in Man: A Critical Review." *Postgraduate Medical Journal* 54 (630): 244–48. https://doi.org/10.1136/pgmj.54.630.244.PMID: 351589; PMCID: PMC2425246.

20. Walker, Alexander R. P. 1972. "The Human Requirement of Calcium: Should Low Intakes Be Supplemented?" *American Journal of Clinical Nutrition* 25 (5): 518–30. https://doi.org/10.1093/ajcn/25.5.518.

21. Heaney, Robert P., Paul D. Saville, and Robert R. Recker. 1975. "Calcium Absorption as a Function of Calcium Intake." *Journal of Laboratory and Clinical Medicine* 85 (6): 881–90. https://pubmed.ncbi.nlm.nih.gov/1138021.

22. Institute of Medicine of the National Academies. 2005. *Dietary Reference Intakes for Energy, Carbohydrate, Fiber, Fat, Cholesterol, Protein, and Amino Acids*. Washington, DC: National Academies Press. https://nap.nationalacademies.org/read/10490.

23. Cheuvront, Samuel N., Robert Carter, and Michael N. Sawka. 2003. "Fluid Balance and Endurance Exercise Performance." *Current Sports Medicine Reports* 2 (4): 202–8. https://doi.org/10.1249/00149619-200308000-00006.

24. Murray, Bob. 2007. "Hydration and Physical Performance." *Journal of the American College of Nutrition* 26 (Sup 5): 542S–548S. https://doi.org/10.1080/07315724.2007.10719656.

25. Kauppila, L. I. 1995. "Can Low-back Pain Be Due to Lumbar-artery Disease?" *The Lancet* 346 (8979): 888–89. https://doi.org/10.1016/s0140-6736(95)92714-x.

26. Kauppila, L. I., A. Penttilä, P. J. Karhunen, K. Lalu, and P. Hannikainen. 1994. "Lumbar Disc Degeneration and Atherosclerosis of the Abdominal Aorta." *Spine* 19 (8): 923–29. https://doi.org/10.1097/00007632-199404150-00010.

27. Wang, Qian, Andrew L. Rozelle, Christin M. Lepus, Carla R. Scanzello, Jason J. Song, D. Meegan Larsen, James F. Crish, et al. 2011. "Identification of a Central Role for Complement in Osteoarthritis." *Nature Medicine* 17 (12): 1674–79. https://doi.org/10.1038/nm.2543.

28. Hajihashemi, Parisa, Leila Azadbakht, Mahin Hashemipor, Roya Kelishadi, and Ahmad Esmaillzadeh. 2014. "Whole-grain Intake Favorably Affects Markers of Systemic Inflammation in Obese Children: A Randomized Controlled Crossover Clinical Trial." *Molecular Nutrition & Food Research* 58 (6): 1301–8. https://doi.org/10.1002/mnfr.201300582.

29. Jiang, Yu, Sheng-Hui Wu, Xiao-Ou Shu, Yong-Bing Xiang, Bu-Tian Ji, Ginger L. Milne, Qiuyin Cai, et al. 2014. "Cruciferous Vegetable Intake Is Inversely Correlated With Circulating Levels of Proinflammatory Markers in Women." *Journal of the Academy of Nutrition and Dietetics* 114 (5): 700–708.e2. https://doi.org/10.1016/j.jand.2013.12.019.

30. VanDenKerkhof, Elizabeth G., Helen M. Macdonald, Gareth T. Jones, Chris Power, and Gary J. Macfarlane. 2011. "Diet, Lifestyle and Chronic Widespread Pain: Results From the 1958 British Birth Cohort Study." *Pain Research and Management* 16 (2): 87–92. https://doi.org/10.1155/2011/727094.

31. Dai, Zhaoli, Jingbo Niu, Yuqing Zhang, Paul Jacques, and David T Felson. 2017. "Dietary Intake of Fibre and Risk of Knee Osteoarthritis in Two US Prospective Cohorts." *Annals of the Rheumatic Diseases* 76 (8): 1411–19. https://doi.org/10.1136/annrheumdis-2016-210810.

Chapter 10

1. Tøien, Tiril, Jakob Lindberg Nielsen, Ole Kristian Berg, Mathias Forsberg Brobakken, Stian Kwak Nyberg, Lars Espedal, Thomas Malmo, Ulrik Frandsen, Per Aagaard, and Eivind Wang. 2023. "The Impact of Life-long Strength Versus Endurance Training on Muscle Fiber Morphology and Phenotype Composition in Older Men." *Journal of Applied Physiology* 135 (6): 1360–71. https://doi.org/10.1152/japplphysiol.00208.2023.

2. MacIntyre, Donna L., W. Darlene Reid, and Donald C. McKenzie. 1995. "Delayed Muscle Soreness: The Inflammatory Response to Muscle Injury and Its Clinical Implications." *Sports Medicine* 20 (1): 24–40. https://doi.org/10.2165/00007256-199520010-00003.

3. Irby, Alyssa, Jacqueline Gutierrez, Claressa Chamberlin, Stephen J. Thomas, and Adam B. Rosen. 2020. "Clinical Management of Tendinopathy: A Systematic Review of Systematic Reviews Evaluating the Effectiveness of Tendinopathy Treatments." *Scandinavian Journal of Medicine and Science in Sports* 30 (10): 1810–26. https://doi.org/10.1111/sms.13734. PMID: 32484976.

4. Benedetti, Maria Grazia, Giulia Furlini, Alessandro Zati, and Giulia Letizia Mauro. 2018. "The Effectiveness of Physical Exercise on Bone Density in Osteoporotic Patients." *BioMed Research International* 2018 (December): 1–10. https://doi.org/10.1155/2018/4840531.PMID: 30671455; PMCID: PMC6323511.

5. Hingorjo, Mozaffer Rahim, Sitwat Zehra, Saima Saleem, and Masood Anwar Qureshi. 2018. "Serum Interleukin-15 and Its Relationship With Adiposity Indices Before and After Short-term Endurance Exercise." *Pakistan Journal of Medical Sciences* 34 (5): 1125–1131. https://doi.org/10.12669/pjms.345.15516. PMID: 30344562; PMCID: PMC6191778.

Chapter 12

1. Sanjana, Faria, Hans Chaudhry, and Thomas Findley. 2017. "Effect of MELT Method on Thoracolumbar Connective Tissue: The Full Study." *Journal of Bodywork and Movement Therapies* 21 (1): 179–85. https://doi.org/10.1016/j.jbmt.2016.05.010.

2. Ockler, Thomas K. 2013. *Muscle Energy Techniques for Pelvis, Sacrum, Lumbar Spine, and Muscles of the Hip*. Lutterworth, UK: AHCS Publishing. https://tomocklerpt.com/product/m1-manual.

3. Burns, Denise K., and Michael R. Wells. 2006. "Gross Range of Motion in the Cervical Spine: The Effects of Osteopathic Muscle Energy Technique in Asymptomatic Subjects." *Journal of Osteopathic Medicine* 106 (3): 137–42. https://pubmed.ncbi.nlm.nih.gov/16585381.

4. Schenk, Ronald, Kimberly Adelman, and John Rousselle. 1994. "The Effects of Muscle Energy Technique on Cervical Range of Motion." *Journal of Manual & Manipulative Therapy* 2 (4): 149–55. https://doi.org/10.1179/jmt.1994.2.4.149.

5. Lenehan, Karen L., Gary Fryer, and Patrick McLaughlin. 2003. "The Effect of Muscle Energy Technique on Gross Trunk Range of Motion." *Journal of Osteopathic Medicine* 6 (1): 13–18. https://doi.org/10.1016/s1443-8461(03)80004-7.

6. Wilson, Eric, Otto Payton, Lisa Donegan-Shoaf, and Katherine Dec. 2003. "Muscle Energy Technique in Patients With Acute Low Back Pain: A Pilot Clinical Trial." *Journal of Orthopaedic and Sports Physical Therapy* 33 (9): 502–12. https://doi.org/10.2519/jospt.2003.33.9.502

7. Selkow, Noelle M., Terry L. Grindstaff, Kevin M. Cross, Kelli Pugh, Jay Hertel, and Susan Saliba. 2009. "Short-Term Effect of Muscle Energy Technique on Pain in Individuals With Non-Specific Lumbopelvic Pain: A Pilot Study." *Journal of Manual & Manipulative Therapy* 17 (1): 14E–18E. https://doi.org/10.1179/jmt.2009.17.1.14e.

8. Ballantyne, Fiona, Gary Fryer, and Patrick McLaughlin. 2003. "The Effect of Muscle Energy Technique on Hamstring Extensibility: The Mechanism of Altered Flexibility." *Journal of Osteopathic Medicine* 6 (2): 59–63. https://doi.org/10.1016/s1443-8461(03)80015-1.

9. Moore, Stephanie D., Kevin G. Laudner, Todd A. McLoda, and Michael A. Shaffer. 2011. "The Immediate Effects of Muscle Energy Technique on Posterior Shoulder Tightness: A Randomized Controlled Trial." *Journal of Orthopaedic and Sports Physical Therapy* 41 (6): 400–407. https://doi.org/10.2519/jospt.2011.3292.

10. Hall, Toby, Ho Tak Chan, Lene Christensen, Britta Odenthal, Cherie Wells, and Kim Robinson. 2007. "Efficacy of a C1-C2 Self-sustained Natural Apophyseal Glide (SNAG) in the Management of Cervicogenic Headache." *Journal of Orthopaedic and Sports Physical Therapy* 37 (3): 100–107. https://doi.org/10.2519/jospt.2007.2379.

11. Konstantinou, K., N. Foster, A. Rushton, and D. Baxter. 2002. "The Use and Reported Effects of Mobilization With Movement Techniques in Low Back Pain Management; a Cross-sectional Descriptive Survey of Physiotherapists in Britain." *Manual Therapy* 7 (4): 206–14. https://doi.org/10.1054/math.2002.0469.

12. Teys, Pamela, Leanne Bisset, and Bill Vicenzino. 2008. "The Initial Effects of a Mulligan's Mobilization With Movement Technique on Range of Movement and Pressure Pain Threshold in Pain-limited Shoulders." *Manual Therapy* 13 (1): 37–42. https://doi.org/10.1016/j.math.2006.07.011.

13. Takasaki, Hiroshi, Toby Hall, and Gwendolen Jull. 2012. "Immediate and Short-term Effects of Mulligan's Mobilization With Movement on Knee Pain and Disability Associated With Knee Osteoarthritis – a Prospective Case Series." *Physiotherapy Theory and Practice* 29 (2): 87–95. https://doi.org/10.3109/09593985.2012.702854.

14. Kim, Sang-Lim, and Byoung-Hee Lee. 2016. "Effect of Mulligan's Mobilization With Movement Technique on Gait Function in Stroke Patients." *Journal of Physical Therapy Science* 28 (8): 2326–29. https://doi.org/10.1589/jpts.28.2326.

15. Hubbard, Tricia J., and Jay Hertel. 2008. "Anterior Positional Fault of the Fibula After Sub-acute Lateral Ankle Sprains." *Manual Therapy* 13 (1): 63–67. https://doi.org/10.1016/j.math.2006.09.008.

16. Bisset, Leanne, Elaine Beller, Gwendolen Jull, Peter Brooks, Ross Darnell, and Bill Vicenzino. 2006. "Mobilisation With Movement and Exercise, Corticosteroid Injection, or Wait and See for Tennis Elbow: Randomised Trial." *BMJ* 333 (7575): 939. https://doi.org/10.1136/bmj.38961.584653.ae.

17. Alkhawajah, Hani A., and Ali M. Alshami. 2019. "The Effect of Mobilization With Movement on Pain and Function in Patients With Knee Osteoarthritis: A Randomized Double-blind Controlled Trial." *BMC Musculoskeletal Disorders* 20 (1). https://doi.org/10.1186/s12891-019-2841-4. PMID: 31627723; PMCID: PMC6800493.

18. Lewis, Cynan, and Timothy W. Flynn. 2001. "The Use of Strain-Counterstrain in the Treatment of Patients With Low Back Pain." *Journal of Manual & Manipulative Therapy* 9 (2): 92–98. https://doi.org/10.1179/jmt.2001.9.2.92.

19. Dardzinski, J. A., B. E. Ostrov, and L. S. Hamann. 2000. "Myofascial Pain Unresponsive to Standard Treatment: Successful Use of a Strain and Counterstrain Technique With Physical Therapy." *Journal of Clinical Rheumatology* 6 (4): 169–74. https://doi.org/10.1097/00124743-200008000-00001.

20. Wong, Christopher Kevin, and Carrie Schauer. 2004. "Reliability, Validity and Effectiveness of Strain Counterstrain Techniques." *Journal of Manual & Manipulative Therapy* 12 (2): 107–12. https://doi.org/10.1179/106698104790825347.

21. Travell, Janet, David Simons, and Lois Simons. 1999. *Myofascial Pain and Dysfunction: The Trigger Point Manual*, 2nd Ed. Baltimore: Lippincott Williams & Williams

22. Simons, David G. 2008. "New Views of Myofascial Trigger Points: Etiology and Diagnosis." *Archives of Physical Medicine and Rehabilitation* 89 (1): 157–59. https://doi.org/10.1016/j.apmr.2007.11.016.

23. Cieslowski, David. 2011. "Trigger Point Therapy. Is It Effective for Pain and Improving Patient Function?" *PT Critically Appraised Topics. Forest Grove, OR: Pacific University*. https://core.ac.uk/download/pdf/48845273.pdf.

24. Nagrale, Amit V., Paul Glynn, Aakanksha Joshi, and Gopichand Ramteke. 2010. "The Efficacy of an Integrated Neuromuscular Inhibition Technique on Upper Trapezius Trigger Points in Subjects With Non-specific Neck Pain: A Randomized Controlled Trial." *Journal of Manual & Manipulative Therapy* 18 (1): 37–43. https://doi.org/10.1179/106698110x12595770849605.

25. Delaney, Joseph P. A., King Sun Leong, Alan Watkins, and David Brodie. 2002. "The Short-term Effects of Myofascial Trigger Point Massage Therapy on Cardiac Autonomic Tone in Healthy Subjects." *Journal of Advanced Nursing* 37 (4): 364–71. https://doi.org/10.1046/j.1365-2648.2002.02103.x.

26. Garfin, S. R., C. M. Tipton, S. J. Mubarak, S. L. Woo, A. R. Hargens, and W. H. Akeson. 1981. "Role of Fascia in Maintenance of Muscle Tension and Pressure." *Journal of Applied Physiology* 51 (2): 317–20. https://doi.org/10.1152/jappl.1981.51.2.317.

27. Lewit, Karel, and Sarka Olsanska. 2004. "Clinical Importance of Active Scars: Abnormal Scars as a Cause of Myofascial Pain." *Journal of Manipulative and Physiological Therapeutics* 27 (6): 399–402. https://doi.org/10.1016/j.jmpt.2004.05.004.

28. Ingber, R. S. 1989. "Iliopsoas Myofascial Dysfunction: A Treatable Cause of "Failed" Low Back Syndrome." *Archives of Physical Medicine and Rehabilitation* 70 (5): 382–386. https://www.archives-pmr.org/article/0003-9993(89)90072-5/abstract.

29. LeBauer, Aaron, Robert Brtalik, and Katherine Stowe. 2008. "The Effect of Myofascial Release (MFR) on an Adult With Idiopathic Scoliosis." *Journal of Bodywork and Movement Therapies* 12 (4): 356–63. https://doi.org/10.1016/j.jbmt.2008.03.008.

30. Liptan, Ginevra L. 2010. "Fascia: A Missing Link in Our Understanding of the Pathology of Fibromyalgia." *Journal of Bodywork and Movement Therapies* 14 (1): 3–12. https://doi.org/10.1016/j.jbmt.2009.08.003.

31. Bedaiwy, M. A., B. Patterson, and S. Mahajan. 2013. "Prevalence of Myofascial Chronic Pelvic Pain and the Effectiveness of Pelvic Floor Physical Therapy." *Journal of Reproductive Medicine* 58 (11–12): 504–510. https://pubmed.ncbi.nlm.nih.gov/24568045.

32. Barnes, John. 1996. "Myofascial Release in Treatment of Thoracic Outlet Syndrome." *Journal of Bodywork and Movement Therapies* 1 (1): 53–57. https://doi.org/10.1016/s1360-8592(96)80016-7.

33. May, Stephen, and Jenny Ross. 2009. "The McKenzie Classification System in the Extremities: A Reliability Study Using Mckenzie Assessment Forms and Experienced Clinicians." *Journal of Manipulative and Physiological Therapeutics* 32 (7): 556–63. https://doi.org/10.1016/j.jmpt.2009.08.007.

34. Clare, Helen A., Roger Adams, and Christopher G. Maher. 2005. "Reliability of McKenzie Classification of Patients With Cervical or Lumbar Pain." *Journal of Manipulative and Physiological Therapeutics* 28 (2): 122–27. https://doi.org/10.1016/j.jmpt.2005.01.003.

35. Machado, Luciana A. C., Chris G. Maher, Rob D. Herbert, Helen Clare, and James H. McAuley. 2010. "The Effectiveness of the McKenzie Method in Addition to First-line Care for Acute Low Back Pain: A Randomized Controlled Trial." *BMC Medicine* 8 (1). https://doi.org/10.1186/1741-7015-8-10.

36. Machado, Luciana Andrade Carneiro, Marcelo Von Sperling De Souza, Paulo Henrique Ferreira, and Manuela Loureiro Ferreira. 2006. "The McKenzie Method for Low Back Pain." *Spine* 31 (9): E254–62. https://doi.org/10.1097/01.brs.0000214884.18502.93.

37. Garcia, Alessandra N., Francine L. B. Gondo, Renata A. Costa, Fábio N. Cyrillo, Tatiane M. Silva, Luciola C. M. Costa, and Leonardo O. P. Costa. 2011. "Effectiveness of the Back School and Mckenzie Techniques in Patients With Chronic Non-specific Low Back Pain: A Protocol of a Randomised Controlled Trial." *BMC Musculoskeletal Disorders* 12 (1). https://doi.org/10.1186/1471-2474-12-179.

Made in the USA
Coppell, TX
29 January 2025